MIND
LOGY

MINDOLOGY

written by

Sushanta Sen

ADHYYAN BOOKS

Mindology

1st Edition

Publication Date: February 2020
Price: ₹ 349 | $ 16.00
ISBN: 978-93-88644-70-9

Published by:

Adhyyan Books
Office No. 637,
Opposite Vivanta by Taj,
DDA SFS. Pocket-1, Dwarka,
Sec-22, New Delhi-110077
Website: http://adhyyanbooks.com
E-mail: contact@adhyyanbooks.com

Dedication

Dedicated to all of you who are passionate to make happiness and success your lifetime-affair in all the domains of life.

Gratefully dedicated to my Mom & Dad, without their blessing I could not have done anything great in my life.

Contents

About the Author *ix*
Acknowledgements *xii*
Foreword (By Dr. M. D. Ray) *xv*
Message *xvii*

1) Prosperous Subconscious Mind 1

2) Relaxation/Meditation 33

3) My True Purpose of Life 41

4) Beautiful Human Body & Sound Health 63

5) Imagination of Magnificent Self-Love & Be a Loving Soul 69

6) Attitude of Gratitude 77

7) Release Emotions through Forgiveness 83

8) Results of a True Relationship 89

9) Effects of Blessings 97

10) Develop a Money-Mindset 101

11) Life without Vision, Goal and Action 105

12) Corporate Hangover 133

13) Major take away from this book 139

14) Exercise 141

About the Author:

Meet Sushanta Sen, your Happiness Coach who has transformed more than two thousand lives and still counting!

Born in a small town in West Bengal Sushanta always dreamed of a happy and successful life since childhood. Today he has not only achieved his dream, he is also helping thousands of others to do the same!

After completing his management studies, he started his corporate journey with a small healthcare company and climbed the corporate ladder slowly and steadily.

It was during his corporate assignments that he became intrigued by and started studying the human mind and its power. "What is next" has always been & continues to be Sushanta's biggest driving force.

He always wanted to contribute positively to society and thus became a life transformation coach.

Toward this mission, he started his own venture "Mindcal Academy" after quitting his job and began researching on human mind and it's potential.

During the last twenty two years of his career he has travelled nineteen countries and studied a wide range of people and their behaviour patterns. He has also explored real secrets of highly successful people and the impact of positive and negative thoughts on the human body. Even today, he devotes four to five hours every day to learn even more about the mind and it's potential.

An entrepreneur who is a very keen learner Sushanta believes that the most effective way to become a master of one's subject is to teach that subject to others so he began teaching & sharing his own knowledge to people around him to empower them with his technical and leadership training program.

During his corporate career Sushanta has conducted numerous life changing workshops for people from varied walks of life.

His purpose in life is:

"To Enrich, Empower and Inspire people to live a healthy, happy and successful life".

Sushanta feels blessed to have gained a deep understanding of the power of human mind through his different Teachers, Gurus, Masters and Mentors. Today he is paying it forward by helping people to understand their lives and empower them to live a vibrant life more happily through his "Mind Power Unlimited" & "Unleash your true Potential" workshops and seminars.

Acknowledgements:

Gratitude:

I want to express my heartfelt gratitude to the following people, who make up my life:

My wife for life and the woman of my dreams, Ruma. You are the most incredible wife, mother and human being I could ever hope to share my life with. With your unwavering support, you make everything I do possible.

My children, Raunak and Soham. You two are my inspiration, and you both mean more to me than anything else in this world.

My sister Susmita and her Children Satarupa and Subhangi for their inspiration in my life.

All of my mentors for their inspiration, motivation and kind support.

A great writer and Dr. M.D.Ray for inspiring me to write a book.

All of my friends, colleagues, and well wishers for their love and critics.

I am really happy and grateful to the editor of this book and the entire team, without their help this book could not be able to come to light this way.

DR (MAJOR) M D RAY
MS, FRCS (UK), FICS (Surg Onco), PhD (Sch, Onco) FAIS, Fellow (Onco Surgery) Senior Research Fellow (Onco Surgery) ICMR, New Delhi"
Addl Prof, Surgical Oncology

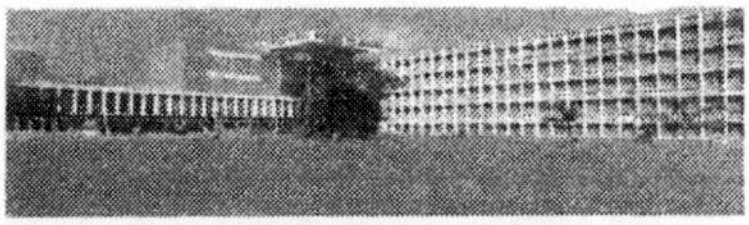

DR BRA INSTITUTE ROTARY CANCER HOSPITAL
ALL INDIA INSTITUTE OF MEDICAL SCIENCES
Ansari Nagar, New Delhi-110029, INDIA
Phone: (O) 011-29575259 Fax: 011-26588641 (O)
M: 9868398339, 9716772975
dr_mdray@yahoo.com, majordrmdray@aiims.ac.in

Foreword:

It gives me immense pleasure to write a foreword for Mr Sushanta Sen's heartful writing the 'Mindology' which is a product of his fifteen years immense study and research, for the entire human beings in this Universe.

Mindology is designed to give the reader a complete understanding of the human mind and its power. The book uses various easy to understand examples which give an in-depth knowledge about how successful people recalibrate, restructure, reengineer and rewire their mind to get the maximum results in their life. This book explains in detail the personality traits needed for a successful life and it also provides you with easy and effective tools, techniques and strategies to develop those traits to create a happy life. It's a practical guide for harnessing the power of our mind and utilizing its potential fully for a joyous & fulfilling life.

I am very much sure that life will have more fulfillments for those who will follow the steps of this book, without any doubt.

Thanking you very much. May the universe bless us together.

Dr. (Major) M D Ray
MS, FRCS (UK), PhD (Onco. Sch.) FICS (Surg. Onco.)
Additional Professor, Dept. of Surgical Oncology
DR. BRAIRCH, AIIMS, New Delhi

Message to all my readers

"The only person you are destined to become is the person you decide to be."

Jack Canfield

One fine morning, when I found myself stuck like a spinning wheel in mud and was cursing my luck, my mother came to me said,"It is only you who can ink the blueprint of your own destiny."Being a broke at that time, I was not convinced by her thought and was sceptical about what my ears were just fed with. I was of an opinion that we are born with a destiny. After my graduation, I ventured into a business,wherein, I failed miserably and was very much hopeless. After that, I spent SIX years sitting at home, doing nothing and struggling with my future career management. I thought my future was buried in a dark tunner and I won't be able to do anything in life. I was eagerly searching for an opportunity.

Eventually, after six years of struggle, I got a chance to pursue my management. I was sure that itwas the only chancc I had tu build my career. I burnt the midnight and scored exceptionally well as per my capability. After completing the management, I was looking for a job and got a chance to serve a healthcare company. I served there for two years and switched over to another big healthcare company. During leadership training, the trainer told all of us that if you want to enjoy your life and want to be successful and happy then you need to understand your mind. That statement triggered my curiosity. Therefore, I decided to research more about the mind and its work.

I visited so many Teachers, Gurus, Masters and Mentors to understand the human mind. I accumulated all the data taught by different masters. I thought of applying all these rules in my life. Slowly and gradually, I started applying all the theories of mind in my real life because I never believe anything until and unless I experience it. Gradually, life started transforming into an amazing journey. I attended countless seminars and workshops conducted by different teachers to understand the function of the human mind. I was only gaining experience and applying the same in my real life.

After witnessing the results, I was convinced that our mind is the only powerhouse in our life and we need to use it very carefully. After realising the fact about mind, I started applying it on different people and they also got the same result which authenticated my claim. I visited many countries and applied the same principal on people from different cultures and mindset and registered the same results. It was anexperiential study I went through and I was completely convinced that these formulas are applicable for everybody if they follow the instruction.

The human mind is like a monkey and so many people compare the human mind with a monkey. It doesn't stay at one single place; it travels much faster than light and sound. I was in the corporate sector for 22 years and in the last 15 years, I have been studying the human mind and its potential. I have used each and every formula on different occasions and received implacable results. I thought that if I can get the tremendous results by applying these formulas then I must spread these success mantras to others.Therefore, I started communicating with people around me, sharing these formulas in my seminars and workshops and they are also convinced that we can get anything we want if we use our mind judiciously.

Thereafter, I started a new venture called Mindcal Academy where I conduct all these workshops and seminars. Our website is **www.mindcal.com** where I have explained our Mission & Vision and what we want to do for people who want to be happy and successful in life. We demonstrate all these formulas in our experiential workshops. I can assure all of you one thing that the way I experience all these methods and their results, you can also fetch the same but the condition applies. And that condition is that you have to practice all these methods for at least NINETY days to make it a habit, as our nature is to stay in our comfort zone.We always prefer to stay at a place and don't want to make any extra efforts to get some outstanding results. "If you are comfortable in any uncomfortable situation then only you can take inspired action." If you practice this formula then you can be comfortable in any uncomfortable situation.You will be empowered to take the inspired action which will cruise you to a place where you feel joy. If you are enjoying your action then you can grow very fast in that direction.

CHAPTER 1

Prosperous Subconscious Mind

Mind is a powerhouse in our life. It gives continuous signals to our body to work continuously without any break. All our five senses receive information from the Universe and send the data to the processing centre to analyze and instruct the body parts to act accordingly. We always misunderstand our mind and its power and hence, we suffer miserably for common reasons.

"Research says that Albert Einstein used only 10% of his Mind. If a scholar like Einstein used 10% then think of a normal person."

We might often wonder why is that:

One person is very successful,whereas, theother fails miserably in life?

One man is meritorious throughout his career but fails in life and another is not good at academics but very successful in life?

One man always incursloss and another is always in profit?

One man is always very healthy and another is always suffering and sick?

One Salesperson is a superstar and another is struggling to survive?

One man is always sad for every reason and another always happy without any reason.

One man is always "lucky" and another always "unlucky"?

One man can heal his or her incurable disease and another cannot heal even a simple cold orcough by oneself?

95% of the wealth in the world is owned by only 1% of people?

We need to think seriously.............

WHAT MAKES FEW INDIVIDUALS MORE SUCCESSFUL THAN OTHERS?

Because only a few have understood "The Subconscious Mind" and "The Principles of Success". Besides, they know

how to use them to create Success, Happiness, Prosperity, Wealth and Good Health in their life!

"Whatever goal you give to the Subconscious mind, it will work night and day to achieve."

Jack Canfield

Successful People have...a big dream...and take inspired action.

They are passionate about their workand don't get tired easily.

They are very much disciplined and methodical.

They are always focusedand do one work at a time.

Their Patience gives them immense power to think and act smartly.

They come forward and always take the responsibility forany adverse outcome.

They always believe in a sense of belongingness and give credit to the team.

They think for themselves,their team members and equally for the society.

They always believe in massive action and they do not procrastinate their work.

They are always calm and cool in any adverse or favourable situation.

They are always visionary and their vision drives them to achieve their goal.

They have never harboured the GIVE UP mentality, they are always persistent and consistent

All these qualities make themtruly ***UNSTOPPABLE...***

In a nutshell, they all know how to use their Mind effectively and efficiently and they are well versed withthe Laws of Success and Law of Universe.

To learn the mechanics of the Human Mind and the Laws of Success,and how to use them to create ***THE LIFE OF YOUR DREAMS***, this book will give you in-depth ideas to make it happen.

There is abundance in this Universe and we can draw from it anything into our life. Universe is like an Ocean. If you take out water in a bucket, it's not going to affect the mighty ocean. However, if we install a Pipeline then we can take as much water with still no deficit to the oceanic body.

You can install a Pipeline into the Ocean of Life i.e. EXPAND our Consciousness level so that you can ferry in whatever you want into your life.

"Consciousness = Knowledge + Understanding"

There are two types of mentality that human beingsharbour. One is ***"SCARCITY"*** mentality and another is ***"ABUNDANCE"*** mentality.

Scarcity is a myth. There is abundance in everything in life.All we need to do is we ought to see from our inner guided system.

Successful people always explore possibilities in any scarcity, and they attract good things in their life.At the same time, Scarcity mentality people fail to see an opportunity even in a favorable situation.

Therefore,we need to open our eyes and ears so that we can sense the opportunity and grab it.We always blame others for our failure andhold others responsible for any consequence.

If we conquer in our mind that.........

I am responsible for my Destiny and Life and I can make my destiny

I will not blame others for any of my failure and adversity.

I will not justify anything in life what so ever it may be.

"Remember, you cannot hire someone to do your push-ups".

If we stop blaming others for any outcome of life and take full responsibility for any outcome, which is directly impacting our life, then 50% of the productivity will improve because we cannot make any excuses for any wrongdoing.

All successful people do follow these three rules all the time. They take 100% responsibility in their life, they don't blame others for any negative outcomes and they never justify anything.

This book will unfurl tothe readers how to use your mind and its highest potential.

There are certain things in life which ONLY YOU HAVE TO DO and for that you have TO BECOME COMFORTABLE WITH BECOMING UNCOMFORTABLE....

We always prefer to stay in the comfort zone and don't explore the possibilities of great success outside it. If we master our selfto handle the uncomfortable in our life, only then we will be comfortable with the uncomfortable.

I know it's easier said than done.

Here, let me share my real story in this context.....

I graduated in business administration and started my career with a basic job. I was doing well and switched over to another company and then again another company. My last assignment was with a Healthcare company and I served there for 8 years three months. Since I was doing thejob of my choice,I was very much comfortable and content. I had been studying the human mind simultaneously for the last 15 years and I was passionate to learn more. It was a great learning experience so far and I was enjoying both of my professions. Life was really beautiful. I never used to look for an option beyond my comfortzone.

Slowly and gradually, I learned to be comfortable in the bubble of my comfort zone. However, after reaching a great height in my career, I felt that my life was boring because I did the same work again and again and there was nothing new to unearth. My creativity started to fade because I could not create anything new.Since I was comfortable,I didn't look around for any other opportunity or explore any new possibilities. I failed several times in my career butI overcame within a short span of time.

I was studying Mind and it's power from 21st May2005. I had been studying and doing research for almost 15 years about the mind and I was applying all the rules on myselffrom time to time to understand the science behind it. I am happy and grateful to all of my Gurus for guiding me and showing me the path for ***REAL*** happiness and success. I tested it several times on different occasions and came to theconclusion that ***MIND CAN BE OUR BEST FRIEND OR THE WORST ENEMY***, souse it properly. I practice certain rituals everyday to know the best performance of my mind. Earlier, I used to work hard and the results were not significant. After using my mind in a positive way, I achieved things thatwere almost impossible. I am so happy and so grateful to the Universe for yielding to me the feelings of abundance in everything. I explored opportunities in the adverse situation and gained out of it. I got my purpose and the answer to why I am here,what I am seeking and what are my expectations. I used all the best possible Mind Tools, Techniques and strategies to achieve my desired goal.

After experiencing the mind and its power, I coach people and help them live happily andsuccessfully.

By following the same practices, even you will be Transformed, you will be Inspired, Motivated and Empowered to achieve anything you desire (any GOAL) and be able to truly live the Life of your dream.

New possibilities will open up for you. Things that seem impossibleto you will become possible.

You will gain awareness of the Laws that govern your life and how you can use these laws for achieving Success, Happiness and Peace of Mind. You will rediscover "Aliveness" in your life.

You will know how to expect major breakthroughs in all areas of your life. If you are stuck in any area of your life because of which you are unable to achieve your GOALS, you will know how to untangle yourself and move forward.

You may expect that you will have all the tools and technologies to become UNSTOPPABLE.

I can Guaranteeyou that after readings this book and taking action, you will root out your problems in all areas of your life.

You have ***"Unlimited Power& Potential"***

Jack Canfield's Success Principle says However, first, you need to take 100% responsibility for yourlife and the results that you produce in your life.

For taking full responsibility, you have to give up 3 things:

- ***Blaming*** others for anything in life
- ***Complaining*** about circumstances,events andpeople
- ***Justifying*** your lack of results and defending your position

AND hold yourself completely ***accountable for your life and the results you produce in your life.***

Jack Canfield's Famous formulais

E + R = O

Event + Response = Outcome

This formula is self-explanatory. Events are not in our hand but the response is always in our hand. Our outcome depends on our Response to any Event. We need to learn the art of response. Response is better than a reactionto any specific situation in our life. We can decide our outcome as per our response. We always blame the events which are bound to come in our life. We face good events and also not so good events. We always expect only good events to transpire in our life but it won't happen because events are not in our control. A proper response to any event is more important. For instance, we always face traffic jam in our city and it creates annoyance within. During these events, different people respond differently. Few fexpress their anger, few feel stressed and few people react patiently to this situation. People who are calm and cool, utilize this time by engaging themselves in a telephonic conversation or listening to educational audios and informationtheir destination about the event. They know that they cannot do much in the present situation and it is better to utilize the situation in a constructive way. On the other hand,there are a few people who are always stressed because of their ignorance. They are unable to understand that they cannot do much and they have to control their negative emotions. Therefore, any event can be utilized differently. Our life is filled with small and big events and we need to face it every day. We need to listen to our inner voice before responding in a particular event.

There are three responses that are very much in our control:

- Our thoughts (self-talk) and beliefs (both conscious and unconscious).

- Our words have a great impact on others. It is not important what we say, it is more significant how we say and behave.
- Our visual imagery during visualization including our images of thefuture.

All you need to learn is: ***MASTERING YOUR THOUGHTS***

Everything is Energy;everything is a Vibration(a frequency).

Law of Attraction says:

Like attracts like. What we give out, we get back. Whatever we put your attention, energy and focus on;we will attract more of the same.

- Thoughts create Feelings, Feelings CreateVibrations and Vibrationhave the potential to Attract

The same rule applies toour Life as well.

Finally, the entire Universe is nothing else but ***VIBRATIONS***.

Our thoughts are very powerful…

Thoughts → Feelings → Vibrations → Attract similar things in your Life

We become what we think about most of the time (dominant thoughts).

We are a product of our thought;our consistent thought about something for a long time would be a reality.

Everything is created twice:

1) First in our mind

2) And, then in the physical world

Law of the Mind: We can CREATE our future by thinking the right Thoughts.Hence,it is said that our thoughts create our destiny.

Research by Dr. Masaru Emoto, Japanese Scientist:

Dr. Emoto has been conducting research on the effect of ideas, words and music upon the molecules of water and he has proven that our thought can change the water quality.

Power of thoughts:

What we are today is because of our yesterday'sthoughts and our present thoughts build our tomorrow's life.

"Our life is the creation of our mind."

- Lord Buddha

"It does not matter where you are coming from, all that matters is where you are going..."

- Frank Turner

Creating the future:

The Point of Power is only in the ***PRESENT MOMENT.***

What you ***THINK, SAY*** and ***DO*** in the ***PRESENT MOMENT*** (the quality of your vibrations in this moment) is what decides your future.

Now, the next question that surfaces is, where do thoughts come from?

Well, they come from our Mind... Simple!

Hence, we need to understand our Mind

So, let'sscuba-dive and understand our Mind:

BRAIN is like the Computer HARDWARE

MIND is like the Computer SOFTWARE

Brain is a tangible part of our body but Mind is intangible. We have two brains:

1) Left Brain

2) Right Brain

The left brain is what we call left Hemisphere or Logical Brain.

Right Brain is the Right Hemisphere or creative brain.

Our Brain has five lobes and eightkinds of intelligence.

Five Lobes are:

Prefrontal, Postfrontal, Parietal,Temporal & Occipital

Eight Intelligence are: INTRA PERSONAL, INTERPERSONAL, LINGUISTIC, LOGICAL, NATURALISTIC, SPATIAL, KINESTHETIC, MUSICAL.

The human mind is very powerful and this is the only difference between the other creatures and the human. We often come across the word Mindfulness that means using the human mind with its full potential. Mind is intangible and only we can use it like the computer software. We are not our mind, mind is just an organ in our body. Research says we can enhance our mind power by practicing different tools, techniques and strategies. When we organize our mind, we get better results. We have to rehearse to get the maximum output from our mind. Mind has certain set principles and we need to understand these principles in the subsequent chapters. We need to understand how to switch-on our mind and how to switch-off our mind. We always switch-on our mind to receive the data for processing in the processing centre which is our mind.After processing the data, mind guides us to take action and this is what produces results. We receive all the information from this Universe through our five senses and send it to our mind for analysis. Our mind processes the data and informs our body parts to take action. As we slowly and gradually understand our mind, we can uncover the power within.

To avoid unnecessary information which will pollute our mind, we need to switch it off. Virus always infiltrates in our mind when we take all the unnecessary information and that information always gets stored in our hardware. These viruses would slow-down the performance of our Mind and it would corrupt the software where the instrumental information is stored. Therefore, we need to quarantine the viruses and format our mind whenever its performance is compromised. We need to restore all the data which isvery important to run our mind and at the same time, we need to delete the unnecessary information. It works like the computer system.

We gathered all the information at the age of THREE and are continuingwith the same informationtill now as nobody told us about the secret of how to delete the unnecessary files. Our hard disk is filled with information we received till now and it will continue till our last breath. Our mind slows down because of this excess data inside it.It'sthe same like a computer which slows down because of too much unwanted data.

To format our mind we must use different tools, techniques and strategies and at the same time by using the same tools, techniques and strategies we restore our important data. It's like filling Nitrogen Air in our tyres where we deflate and inflate at the same time. So, on one side, we remove all the negative things stored in our mind and all the new positive things can be installed simultaneously. Our mind is a receptor that receives all the information from our five senses. All our five senses are like catalyststhat just pass the data to our mind.Our mind, then, instructs our five senses and the whole body to respond as per the situations,circumstances and events.The results and response dependon our mind's programming. It can react or respondto the same situation, circumstance and people. It depends on our mind's programming to understand the situation, circumstance or people to react or respond.

Events or circumstances are not in our control but the response in that circumstance or event is in our control. We always want to control the events and circumstances which is not possible and due to this, we take wrong decisions. Sometimes the unpleasant situation and circumstances are inevitable and the smart and successful people simply switch-off their mind instantly to avoid any type of escalation of that situation. All successful people know all these secrets of mind and they know very well how to organize and calibrate their mind.

I have interviewed several successful people and have observed one thing that they use their mind in a certain way knowingly or unknowingly. I have even talked to several less-educated people and found them very successful because they use their mind through the tools techniques and strategies unknowingly.When I asked them how they came to know about these tools, techniques and strategies, they simplysaid that they don't know but they have been using all these every time. At the same time, I interviewed educated successful people and they said that they have been trained by the experts,they use it as per the recommendation and have been getting unbelievable results. It has been observed that by using the mind's power, anyone can accomplish anything. All successful people know this formula and they have become unstoppable. If we can understand our mind then we can achieve our goal. We call our mind a monkey mind because it is very difficult to control and the mind travels faster than light and sound. To control our mind is an art as well as science.

We have Two Minds:

1) ***CONSCIOUS MIND***

2) ***SUBCONSCIOUS MIND***

Our conscious mind is like the tip of the Iceberg and the subconscious mind is like the underwater portion of the Iceberg.

Now let's us talk about the powers of these.

Two Minds…

Power of the Conscious Mind

CONSCIOUS MIND is like ALADDIN…

The conscious mind can think; it is called the Logical Mind or Watchman(analyzing, judging, applying logic,and reasoning). The conscious mind takes decisions and action. It can identify and Seize Opportunities. It is called Intelligence Quotient (IQ)

SUBCONSCIOUS MIND is like GENIE…

It has the ability to Attract.It is the Creator of people, events, opportunitiesand ideas to fulfill your wishes.

It's our Inner Guidance System.

Creative Mind, Infinite Intelligence, WisdomEQ and SQ.

It's like a hard Disk with unlimited space. All Past experiences and Beliefs are stored here(subconscious patterns, sanskaras)

The Subconscious Mind is very powerful. If guided correctly by our Conscious Mind, we can use the Subconscious Mind to achieve any Goal and solveany problem. It has 90% of the power. It's like a fertile land where whatever seed you sow, it has the immense power to convert that seed into a full-grown tree. If we sow an apple seed, it will grow apple and if we sow an orange seed, it will grow orange. It will not ask any question. It's like the divine power, it will convert the thought into reality.It cannot make out whether we are imaging or it'sa reality. Most of the people in this universe are unaware of the power of our subconscious mind.

Whatever you can impress on your Subconscious Mind, you can express in your Life

UNIVERSAL LAW: ***AS YOU SOW, SO SHALL YOU REAP***

Conclusion:"What we think we become."– Buddha

What we BELIEVE, we will see in our Life.

So, if you believe:

- The Market is slow, Competition is too tough, Target is too difficult to achieve
- This disease (Diabetes, Cancer, Heart Problems) is not curable
- No one cares for me, No one appreciates me
- I am not good enough, I don't have that flair in me, I am not intelligent
- Life is too difficult, I have to work very hard to earn money

- Men are dominant, Mother-in-laws are bad
- The world is not safe, People always take advantage of me

The same will become true for you...

Now, the Choice is ours, should we continue to water these Negative, Disempowering Beliefs or have Positive, Empowering Beliefs...

Power: In short, if we Program our Subconscious Mind correctly, we can Achieve Anything*

*Conditions apply – ***PROVIDED THERE IS A BURNING DESIRE*** and100% BELIEF in yourself and your GOAL;the *"**Why**"* Of your Life. Knowing why you are here is more important and if you know WHY you are here then the HOW will iron out automatically. We all have experienced our Subconscious MIND one day or the other but are unable to understand the how. Sometimes we think of somebody and that person calls at the same time. If we Experience what we want with feelings, then the Universe conspires to give it to us. We always experience all these events in our life but we are unable to understand why and how it is happening.

We know some power is there which we callas the Divine power but actually it's our Subconscious power. We need to understand our subconscious mind completely and it's potential. I will explain more on this in the subsequent chapters. We can control our subconscious mind by using different tools techniques and strategies. If we understand our subconscious mind properly then we can control it to a great extent.

If we practice the tools, techniques and strategies regularly then we can control our subconscious mind. Successful people always use their subconscious mind to achieve their goals. They know that they have immense power and it lies in their subconscious mind. They use this power every day. I interviewed a few successful people and observed that they don't know the science behind it but have been using their subconscious mind in everything and they are achieving their goals. When I explain to them that there is a science behind it,theyfeel astonished that they have been using their subconscious mind for a long time and they didn't know anything about it. We are being conditioned everyday by our parents, family members, friends, neighbor and peers and that goes to our subconscious mind because the repetition of words can reach our subconscious mind easily. At the age of 3-8, our conscious mind which we call logical mind doesn't apply logic in everything.That's why it is being suggested that during this age, we should notfeed out mind with negative words. During this age group,the subconscious mind picks up all the good or bad things; it cannot differentiate the good things and bad things at all. We are often instructed that we must give good ***SANSKAR***(ethics) to the children so that it goes to their subconscious mind directly. If we put negative words or thoughts in children's mind then it would be stored immediately in their subconscious mind because their conscious mind/Logical mind doesn't put logic to the thoughts or words. Till the age of 8 years, all this mind-conditioning is done and it is stored in their hard disk forever. This programming cannot be deleted easily because it is stored in the subconscious mind and that conditioning makes those children behave like they do.

Our subconscious mind acts as per the data stored inside it. At the age of 3-8,we, as parents/elders, need to be extra careful while using words. Our childhoods were conditioned so deeply that it takes a long time to recondition or recalibrate our mind. It is very much possible to deprogramour mind by using the mind power tools, techniques and strategies. It again depends upon the level of the thoughts stored in the subconscious mind. Our subconscious mind is our powerhouse and we need to choose the proper positive commands to reset it. Subconscious mind cannot identify a positive or negative command, it only implements the command and bring all the people, circumstances and events to our life as per the command sent to it. We can train our subconscious mind through "self-talk". When we repeat the words every time then our subconscious mind can take that command without any logic. We can reach our subconscious mind indifferent ways but we need to allow our conscious mind to sleep and then we can go deep down to our subconscious mind. We need to go to the Alpha level of consciousness and give the command to our subconscious mind. To reach the natural alpha stage,there are two times of the day that are considered ideal; once when you wake up in the morning and when you retire to sleep. We can program our subconscious mind naturally in these two times.

As we read in the beginning that 90% of is power lies with our subconscious mind and 10% with our conscious mind. If we communicate with our subconscious mind properly then we can achieve our goal and accomplish success in our life. There is always a link between us and our subconscious mind. We need to establish the connection all the time so that whatever decision we take is right in our life and we can achieve our desired goal. We know that desire is the seed of any creation and we need to send our message of desire to our subconscious mind to convert it into reality. The subconscious mind cannot differentiate that the picture is an imagination or a reality. If we imagine anything then also it will assume that it's a reality and it will bring all the people, circumstances and events to our life which will make it a reality. We have to dream big and put our subconscious mind to work. It will create all the possible steps to reachour dream but at the same time, our logical or conscious mind has to identify the opportunity so that we can grab success.

We have to chase our goal by taking massive action. "Action without a goal is haphazard anda Goal without action is merely a wish". We need to ignite our subconscious mind which can take care of everything in our life. To ignite it, we need to understand the trigger point and it depends upon our understanding about it. It is our subconscious mind thatcan give us the intuitive power and helps us in developingour sixth sense. Intuitive power is the most important aspect of our subconscious mind which can be developedby using the tools, techniques and strategies. There is a saying, "Practice makes man perfect" and it is well-tested. Any new thing that we need to adapt to will take sometime but if we do it continuously, consistently and persistently then it will give us our desired results. We learn Bicycle riding and Car driving within a certain time. Initially, we take the pain to learn it but few of us give up in between and their logical mind comes in-between and they quit. However, once you have learned,it stays there in your subconscious forever. In the same way, if we practice the tools, techniques and strategies on a regular basis, we can learn to give command to our subconscious mind. We have to put all these techniques, tools and strategies in our DNA,only then we can live with it. All these practices will help us to activate our inner guided system. It's like the GPS system. Our Inner guided system will guide us to reach our goal. It will bring circumstances, people and events to us and guide us from time to time about what to do and what not to do.

We experience this quite often, as we desire for a certain outcome, we come across people who guide us to achieve our goal easily. In our day-to-day life if we have a burning desire to accomplish anything then it will come to us, however, we need to recognize the opportunities with our Conscious mind and seize those immediately. Sometimes we ignore the message from our subconsciousand hence, we fail to recognize the opportunity. All successful people know their subconscious very well.Therefore, they recognize opportunities very easily and seize them. Our intuitive power is inside us but we do not know how to ignite it. If we practice all these techniques then our intuitive power would be enhanced. We can increase our intuitive power by calming down our mind. Through Breathing exercise and Meditation we can help our mind to calm down and we can enhance the intuitive power. Whenever our mind is calm, our intellect awakes,this Intellect gives us the direction to take any decision wisely and achieve our goals. Our subconscious reprogramming can remove our negative belief system and install a new positive belief system. We were programmed during our childhood and we have been carrying that the same belief system till now.This limiting belief system is what holds us back fromtakinge any new decision which is not stored in our hard disk. If any new positive circumstance surfacesin our life,we just ignore it because our belief system does not believe in those positive circumstances.

Our old belief system drives us and we are not aware of it.This old belief system is so deep-rooted that even if our sensory organs recognize any opportunity or circumstances, it will be simply rejected by our subconscious mind. We close our sensory organs to recognize it. Our childhood programming is so intense that it drives us to a certain direction and does not allow us to explore any new things happening in and around us. It's very difficult to reprogram our subconscious mind and to do it we need to rewrite the program. It's a continuous process that demands a lot of patience and never-give-up attitude because the improvement is very slow and we are not consistent. We easily give up in between because of the lack of patience. We want quick results like the Allopathic medicine. We don't have the patience to explore any alternative medicine. It is a very slow process and all the garbage cannot be thrown out of our mind so easily because out mind perceives it as reality. It has been seen that only 10% of people are able to reprogram their subconscious mind because of its slow movement.However, it's very much possible to rewire our subconscious mind. To re-engineerour subconscious mind, we have to commit our self to connect to our subconscious mind regularly without fail. Our connections can be broken frequently in the initial stage but as we progress, it will stay connected whenever we want. We have to develop ourselves to connect with our subconscious mind instantly and we can stay with it as long as we want without any signal drop. We can create our destiny by reprogramming our subconscious mind. Our destiny depends on our childhood programming. We can exploit our subconscious mind and get a magnificent outcome thatwe have never thought of. "Life is Beautiful" and we need to experience this. Our subconscious mind is responsible for our life. It guides us to take decisions and actions. In our life, we procrastinate most of our desires and actions. Procrastination is a disease and to overcome this disease we have to be goal-oriented and every day we need to monitor the progress.

One of India's great teachers and our former President Dr.Abdul Kalam Sir quoted"Dream is not that which you see while sleeping, it is something that does not let you sleep."We need to break this procrastination cycle so that our goal chases us and we are motivated to take action always. We can't afford to linger on any action by hurling excuses. Procrastination is a mental state which stops us to from taking action and achieving our goals. We have to break this state by taking small action everyday for a particular goal. Our subconscious sends us ideas everyday but we are unable to catch them because we don't know how to store them. It hatches new ideas but our conscious mind doubts on it and it goes off. Idea-generation is the creation of our subconscious mind. We need to monitor all the ideas on a regular basis and it's better to store in a note pad so that it won't be misplaced. We need to review all these noted ideas everyday at the end of the day andexplore the possibilities to take it to the analysis level. Our Subconscious mastery depends upon our action taken to bring it back to our life. We are powerful and it was very well visible in our childhood when we were not conditioned by our surroundings.But that power has become dormant because of other's influence on us and we believe it as reality. We are the servant of our subconscious mind rather than our Subconscious mind being our servant. We need to awaken the Genie within and give the command to achieve our desired goal. It will help us by bringing the people, circumstances and events to our life and give us the opportunity to recognize it and act on it so that we can easily achieve our desired goal.

To access our Subconscious mind, we need to go to the Alpha state of consciousness and give command.This command will go straight to our subconscious mind and we would be able to listen to our inner voice which will navigate us to accomplish our desired demand. We need to listen to our inner voice carefully and it will give us thsolutions which can manifest in our life.

Our subconscious mind cannot forget anything because the hard disc capacity is boundless and it can store any amount of data. As explained earlier,since our childhood we have been storing data in our subconscious mind. We can check our subconscious mind easily. Whenever any event comes in our later stage of life and if the same thing happened in our childhood then we can recall it easily. It shows that the past is already stored in our subconscious mind which is triggered now when the same thing repeats in our life. We have experienced it several times in our life through our five sensory organs. We receive the information from our five senses,process it in our mind and take action as per our logical mind. Why we are unable to delete any information and feelstuck is because we hold it like it is a permanent event which is not true.We don't release it and by chattering the same thing again and again, it moves towards our subconscious mind. We take all the grudges and it affects our life. It's very easy to say to remove the events from our life but very difficult to do because our mind is conditioned in such a way that any event seems to be permanent.

However, spiritual practices like Pranayam, Meditation and Relaxation are the proven tools to keep your mind calm and cool and remove all the garbage from your mind. Scientific tools are available to remove all these emotions which are stored in our hard disk. Actually, we need to rewrite our hard disk. All these emotional viruses have corrupted the software and mind with a virusand hence, our mind cannot work with its full potential.How have these viruses entered our mind? It comes through our five senses whenwe take everything without analyzing the information that contains the virus. The sorting of information is very much required before sending it to our subconscious mind for storage. Our analytical mind applies logic every time but is unable to restrict thoughts from entering our subconscious mind. The thoughts which are negative and give us stress would also enter our subconscious mind. Therefore, we need to monitor our thoughts and it can be developed by spiritual practices. We need to bring our mind back to the present moment.

If we accept the thoughts and allow them to pass on then after sometimes the intensity and the number of thoughts would be less. Research says that we can reprogram our subconscious mind through different tools, techniques and strategies. Our mind is like a monkey which is running here and there every moment. We have to slow it down by breathing exercises. Our breath can only control our mind. Be aware of all the thoughts and analyze thembefore sending them to the subconscious mind. As mentioned earlier, repetition of thoughts can easily enter our subconscious mind. There is always a link between our five senses, conscious mind and subconscious mind. Our network should be so strong that the link should be established within a second. It can be like the inverter backup, when the power fails, it switches over to inverter and gives uninterrupted power. Our antenna has to be so strong that it can receive any weak signal very easily. Opportunity is always there around us but we fail to recognize it due to our stressful mind.

Our subconscious mind is always connected to infinite intelligence but we have viruses thatwon't allow us to connect to the source. We have to install a strong antivirus to protect our mind from the virus attack. Strong anti-viruses are available and these tools, techniques and strategies can put a very powerful antivirus in place to protect from a possible attack. We always envelop ourselves in doubts and these doubts harm us from taking action in our life. Our logical mind spawns doubts very often and it doesn't allow us to take action. Doubts are the killer of our big achievements and it comes from our conscious mind. Our past conditioning plays a vital role inweaving the doubts. We have been carrying our past beliefswhich were installed during our childhood. There is a saying that "Faith can move mountains" and it's very much true. Faith is the biggest strength ofour life. Because of our past belief system we do have a lack of faith in everything and always thinkthat it is not possible. Possibilities are there in everything and we don't see it with our preoccupied mind. We have to analyze the possibilities in every moment of our life. Our Subconscious mind is like the motor of th fan. When we put heavy pressure on the fan by runningit without break then the motor can blow up and we need to rewire the motor. The same case happens to our mind, when we don't give rest to it, it just blows off and we need to rewire our mind to get the optimum results again.

CHAPTER 2

Relaxation/Meditation

Meditation is the only food for mind. We need to learn meditation and practice it every day without fail. Regular practice of Meditation can give us clarity. If we are irregular in Meditation then we cannot expect good results. Even FIVE minutes of regular meditation is ok if we can't spare more time. We need to increase the duration slowly and gradually. In the initial stage, it's very difficult to meditate but one needs to sit regularly even if he/she is unable to focus on the thoughts. The only thing to observe is Breath. Our mind moves here and there very fast. We cannot hold it even for a second. According to a research, every day we receive 60000 – 90000 thoughts and most of our thoughts are negative. It's a chain of thoughts sometimes. One thought manifests other thoughts and it goes on. Our thoughts create feelings and feelings create vibrations; we send these vibrations to the Universe and whatever we send out will come back to us. That's why whenever we send negative thoughts, we receive negative vibrations from the Universe. We are the creator of our life as Buddha said,***"We are what we think"***. Meditation is the only tool thatcan calm down our mind and our intellect can be awakened. An agitated mind cannot be productive,rather our life can turn into a mess because of agitation.

Our intellect awakes whenever our mind is calm and cool. There is a big difference between Prayer and Meditation. Whenever we talk to God for anything then it is a prayer but when God talks to us then it's called Meditation. Meditation is being explained by different masters in different ways. We can practice it in a very simple way. Meditation depends upon practice. It's a very old practice to bring our mind back to the present moment. We always think about our past and worry about our future. We always suffer a lot because of our Past and Future. We need to Practice, Practice and Practice Meditation everyday without fail. Meditation can bring back our focus and enhances our intellect to do every work intelligently. During the morning time before the sunrise and before going to bed we can sit quietly with our eyes closed and observe our breaths. Initially,it's very difficult to close our eyes even for 1 minute but as we practice it regularly it will enhance with the passage of time. Whatever thoughts come we need to welcome and let it go. This practice will increase the stability and time of meditation. It's everybody's Endeavour to keep the mind calm and cool but very difficult to do. Consistency is the key to get the best result. Consistent effort will help us focus on meditation. If we leave it in between then it won't be effective.In ancient times, all our sages used to do Meditation practices. The same practices are now being spread by all the masters all across the globe. Our ancient mythology also tells us the same thing. Meditation is a way to make our mind aware of everything in life. All the successful people do it regularly and it's their routine.

Factually, our mind can do only a single work at a time. However, we always do multi-tasking and that's why we are unable to finish a particular task within a certain time. Our life is full of adventures and we don't enjoy these adventures because we are stuck somewhere else. Meditation can rule out our problems in life. It takes a lot of time to bring back our true self because we were programmed in our childhood and our beliefs are very deep-rooted. Our belief system is responsible for our stagnation in life because we don't even try to explore any new things and are always surrounded bythe fear of losing something. We are working in a set protocol and we don't work against the protocol. Meditation is the only tool which can realign our mind. We always curse our self for anything in life but never want to understand the problems. We need to do self-talk and positive affirmation all the time in our life. We are the slave of our mind and we need to make it happy as our masters do. We always think that mind can't do everything because we do not know the power of our mind and it's potential. Meditation is a very simple and Meditative state that can be developed over a period of time. It's a very simple process to start.Initially, it looks odd to you because the feeling is different and you never experienced it before.

Relaxation is very much required to slow down our mind. Our mind is very hyperactive and always travels here and there. As we can control with proper breathing, we have to practice proper breathing practices which are very simple.Regular practice of these processes will develop into a habit. Our life is totally depending upon our mind and we need to take very well care of it. Morning practices will generate excellent results because the Nature is cool at that time and the energy is very high in and around us. Sages in ancient India always stressed upon Meditation and relaxation to be in the present moment. The present moment can be achieved if we follow our breath. We can change our breathing pattern by practice. If we breathe very slowly then it will bring back our mind in the present moment. The present moment is the only powerful moment. It is the present moment that decides our future but we are always worried about the future and ignore our present moment. Only practice can bring us to the present moment.

Take a long deep breath, hold it for ten seconds and release it fully. Meditation will remove agitation from your mind. All successful people doself-introspection through meditation. Our inward journey will make us feel aware of our inner being. Our inner voice is very much powerful and it is only the subconscious mind thatgives us instruction through the inner voice. We can do this practice in the morning or evening on an empty stomach so that mind cannot be disturbed. If our stomach is full with food then we cannot concentrate and thoughts will bother us. Many years back our ancestors used to follow the "Early to bed and Early to rise" principal which made them energetic, vibrant and disease-free. Actually, in the morning, the energy is very high and the environment is silent which does not disturb our mind. The external sound also affects our internal sound. If the external sound is high then we cannot listen to our internal sound.When the mind is calm and relaxed then we can listen to our internal sound or inner voice. We always hear our sixth sense when our mind is calm and cool and the sixth sense is none other than our inner voice. Our sixth sense guides us properly and cannot give us a wrong signal. However, we do not have time to listen to our inner voice and hence, we miss the signals. We always prefer to listen to the outside of our body and react to it but the answer toany question comes from within. Our tendency is to look around but not within. We are the slave of our thoughts and we need to monitor our thoughts. If we can manage to do so then we can live happily. Happiness is a choice. We need to choose our thoughts to be happy and let go the unnecessary thoughts. It can be done by observing thoughts during meditation.

I have interviewed many people so far and the rule is the same for everybody. It's a rule of thumb and all successful people know the fact very well.They can monitor their thoughts and take action on their positive thoughts. Positive thoughts come for a little time and if we can continue with these for a long time then it becomes a habit. Ideas come to us very frequently but we cannot hold it for a long time;it vanishes and never comes back. All the successful people write down their each and every idea and scrutinize them from time to time to explore the possibilities. One idea can change our life.

The famous inventor Thomas Edison invented the bulb because of his idea of creating it and it got stuck to his mind. The ten thousand failureswerehis biggest example of consistent efforts.WrightBrother's idea was to create a machine thatcan fly and they invented the Airplane.They must have failed several times but their idea turned into reality. Ideas come to our mind when our mind is cool and calm and thoughtless. Meditation can relax our mind and we can generate new ideas. We do not hold or pen down our ideas for further exploration. Ideas are the richest assets of all the successful people and they do not waste it. They know that one idea can make the fortune and they monitor all the ideas coming to their mind to explore the possibilities to make fortune. Ideas to fortune have so many ups and downs which can be tolerated firmly. All the successful people take this challenge as adventure and romance with it.Their romance is so intense that they just live with it until and unless they get the result. Only an idea can transform into physical reality. This transformation happens when massive action is taken against that idea. Ideas can be anything thatseems impossible but when the action is taken a miracle happens.Meditation is the only medicine for our mind to generate ideas. Our inner voice gives us the signal to act on a certain thing and if we ignore it then it goes forever.

CHAPTER 3

My True Purpose of Life

Understanding Life's Purpose

We all have a Purpose for being on this Planet…We all have a ROLE to play…

Each one of GOD's creation has aPurpose, nothing is extra.

We have been created for a definite purpose.

To play this role, we have been given special talents, qualities and abilities.

Remember that we are all unique and special creations of GOD…No one else can be like you and no one can fulfill your role...

In fact, everything GOD creates is unique.

Living life with a Purpose

Once we understand what we are meant to do and start living "With a Purpose", life becomes extraordinary, easy and joyfulbecause that's what you are meant to do.

You are full of energy and work is no longer work. The Universe **supports you** in all the possible ways.

"JOY" is the measure of how much you aligned ***"With the PURPOSE"***

"Definiteness of purpose is the starting point of all achievement."

– W. Clement Stone

Discovering the Life's Purpose. How to Discover your Life's Purpose? You can discover your life's purpose by reflecting on your 'special skills and talents' and activities that give you maximum JOY.Generally, these activities always involve making a difference inother people's lives.

In our lifetime,most of us are unable to find out our real purpose. We are not at all happy with the work we are doing but due to family pressure, obligation and pressure for the survival we are doing the job. In our childhood, we were programmed for our career and we had chosen our career as per our family and the neighbor. We could not explore our purpose because nobody in the school has taught us about how to know our real purpose in this life.

After a certain age, we are not satisfied with our job and it becomes boring. We are not aware ofhow to know the purpose of life. We have not realized that one big GENIE is staying inside us and is always eager to know what we want in life. Our ***GENIE*** is always ready and tells us ***"YOUR WISH IS MY COMMAND".*** However, we don't know how to awaken the ***GENIE***. All successful people know this secret science and they always use this science to achieve their goal. All successful people know their purpose and they are fully energetic and alert all the time. They never miss the opportunities and grab it as soon as it comes to their life. They are always on their purpose.

By asking our subconscious mind in the Alpha state of consciousness, we can explore:

What is our life's purpose?

What is our unique role in this Universe?

The answer will be given to us directlyor through some events happening in our Life but we need to identify it immediately after it pops up

Nowadays scientific tools are there to find out your Natural Intelligences,skills and talents that are ***GOD GIFTED.***

Purpose of life: What is our ***REAL PURPOSE*** on this planet?

It is to ***SERVE OTHERS*** by making use of our ***UNIQUE*** talents and abilities.

Life's purpose statement by different successful people in this Universe:

"To inspire and empower people to achieve their destiny."

– Robert Allen

"To create and inspire one million millionaires who each gives $ 1 million to their church as charity."

– Mark Victor Hansen

"To inspire and empower people to live their highest vision in context of love and joy."

– Jack Canfield

"My purpose is to Enrich, Empower and Inspire people to live their life happily and successfully".

"What" do I truly want?If we want wealth, then we need clarity in terms of quantity like 1 million dollars within a fixed date. Clarity is power and Clarity rewires our mind.

If you fail to plan your life, you plan to fail...

Power of clarity:

The Number ONE reason why people don't get what ***they want in their Life is that they don't know what they want in their Life.***They don't have clarity and they mess up everything and their action is also not focused because of the lack of clarity.

"The only person you are destined to become is the person you decide to be."

– Ralph Waldo Emerson

Awakening the Genie:

Have 100% Clarity of what you want to BE, DO and HAVE.

This is necessary to trigger the Inner GPS system.

Be 100% clear of WHAT YOU WANT (What do you want to BE, DO and HAVE?)

CLARITY = POWER and IT IS THE TRUTH

Our subconscious mind likes clarity. For example,if you command to your subconscious mind that I want wealth then it will be confused.But if you tell that I want one million rupees salary every month from a certain date like 1st April 2020 then the subconscious will take the command and bring events, circumstances and people to your life to make it a reality. Once the command is accepted by the subconscious mind then it will fulfill your demand as early as possible.However, at the same time, our conscious mind has to identify the opportunity and seize it instantly. Our subconscious mind is always awake but our logical mind obstructs the logic and won't allow a thought or command to reach our subconscious mind. If you can manage to bypass it then the thoughts or commands can reach directly to the subconscious mind. All successful people know how to bypass their conscious mind. The subconscious mind has intuitive power and it sends out the message to the Universe.It brings all the circumstances, events and people to your life to make it happen. It has immense potential and it can bring anything in your life. It's a secret and successful people use their subconscious mind knowingly or unknowingly. I have met many successful people on different occasions and have interviewed them.I observed one thing is common that they use their subconscious mind knowingly or unknowingly.They admitted that they have intuitive power and always receive information through their intuitive power and that's what makes them different from the crowd. Most of them are from the rags to riches category. They know their Genie and their commands are easily accepted. All powers are there within and to understand that we need to understand our subconscious mind completely. Anybody can access their subconscious mind if he or she has a burning desire. Burning desire is like you cannot sleep peacefully until and unless you connect to your subconscious mind.

All ideas come from our subconscious mind only but we ignore it without exploring it further. Ideas can be a reality if we take action and seize the opportunity. Seizing opportunity is also an art because the subconscious mind will give us the signal and if you miss it once then it is gone forever. The signals are very subtle and a person won't take it seriously. Our subconscious mind gives us a clue and our conscious mind has to seize it immediately. Both the minds have to be aligned so that the opportunities can be grabbed instantly. Successful people always see an opportunity in their failure and they use their subconscious mind wisely to explore the opportunity. Our Subconscious mind shows us the route and the route is full of adventures. People easily give up because they don't want to explore the adventures and always want to be in a comfortable position. I have seen people's journey nothing less than a roller coaster ride but one thingthat is common among all the successful peopleis that they never give up. A classic example is Thomas W. Edison who is the inventor of lamp. He failed 10000 times before the invention and he was so sure that he will invent it after so many failures. He had a great belief and faith in himself. There is a saying, "Faith can move mountains" is true for all those who have failed miserably and bounced back with great success. Research says that a calm and cool mind can think wisely and it has great intuition to attract what they want. ***HOW*** is not tough when your ***WHY*** is clearly defined. Inspiring 'why'can put you into action mode and Inspiredaction makes you enlightened. Your energy would be high for Inspiring action and you will not feel tired.

Generally, there are two types of actions; one is ***OBVIOUS ACTION*** and another one is ***INSPIRED ACTION.*** When we are in a joyful state to perform any action then we must know that the action is inspired action. Our subconscious gives us a signal of our ***WHY*** and if we work on our ***WHY*** we can reach our destination without much resistance. Our subconscious mind is responsible to draw the power from the infinite intelligence for us. It is our power to be awakened and make a difference in this Universe. We are here on this planet for a certain period of time and if we make some little difference on this planet then we are really blessed.To make a difference in people's life on this planet, we need to understand the power of our Subconscious and make ourself powerful so that we can achieve our goal. All inventors start with an idea andturn it into reality by the power within. Ideas come when the mind is calm and cool and our subconscious is activated. There are scientific researches which say that if anyone is rag to rich then they are the master of their life. They have self-mastery and they have the winner's mentality. They have the courage to face failure and they know how to bounce back in life. If they are out of track then they can realign themselves to be on track. Subconscious mind is always eager to listen to your command and execute that command. Our conscious mind always puts logic in between and won't allow it to happen. We have different routes to reach our subconscious mind and give the command for execution or results. Our subconscious mind is like the GPS system which guides us to reach our destination. Subconscious mind is our inner guided system which tells us about the route to our destination. It will guide usto the events, circumstances and people to follow. It will guide you where to take the right turn, where to take the left turn and where to take A U-turn.

"We are born with a purpose, not by accident".

Everybody on this planet has a purpose and we spend our entire life to understand the same but are still unable to find it. The famous singer Ms. LataMangeskar had a purpose that she followed and she has been a famous singer since last four decades. Similarly, the cricket legend, Sachin Tendulkardefined his purpose during is childhood.He always dreamed of cricket and he always thought of cricket. Some people understand their purpose at a very early stage and some people spend their whole life to unearth their purpose. Actually, we are conditioned during our childhood.We choose our purpose as per our influencer and struggle in our life.Most of the time we are influenced by our surroundings and flow with their suggestion. We are unable to find our purpose because of the pressure generated by people around us. Every life has a purpose and we have to understand our purpose.

We can find our definite purpose by observing our love and joy. It's our inner messageand we need to explore our purpose by listening to our inner self. If we enjoy any of the tasks we do fully and emotionally then that could be thepurpose of our life. Purpose can be more than one but with similar work. Like if anyone's purpose is to play music and spread happiness to others then he or she can be a music director, composer and a music instrument playerwhile also being a singer.

If the purpose is explored at an early stage then the achievement can be awesome. If we are on a purpose then our effort would be less to achieve that purpose. If we are not on our purpose then we have to put all our efforts and the results don't come easily as per our expectations.

As I elaborated that the only difference between humans and animals is the intellect. We can think and take decisions. Every human being is born with mind and everybody is unique in their behavior pattern. We can observe our purpose by observing the joy and bliss in our life. We are very well connected with the source and if we break the connection then we could not find our purpose. We have to observe our life from the beginning and see which action in our life gives us joy. If the Joy is consistent and continuous then we can decode our purpose. If the joy is not consistent and continuous then it is a temporary joy. Permanent joy in any action or work is our purpose. If we find our purpose in the later stage then we need to groom our purpose without affecting the current work and reacha certain level to quit the current job. Therefore, always search for your purpose sincethe work becomes effortless if he or she is living with apurpose.

"Our Body Organs have a definite purpose"

Each and every organ of our body is meant for a definite purpose. We have major body organs like Liver, Heart, Kidney, Pancreas, etc. All our body organs are working 24/7 X 365 days. The heart is meant for pumping blood,itdoes not get exhausted even for a millisecond or that could prove to be the last second of our life. It started pumping blood when we were in our mother's womb and is still pumping blood. It never asks for rest. Can we afford to give rest to our heart for a second? No....... then we need to go to the life support system to live. So the purpose of our heart is to pump blood,it doesn't get tired even for a single second and is enjoying its job. Same is the case with our another significant organ Liver. It always detoxifies our body and it is doing constantly and consistently. Similar ways our Kidney is meant to filter out the toxin from our body and it is doing continuously and consistently. The pancreas are meant for producing insulin and it regulates the blood sugar level in the body. If it doesn't produce insulin then the blood sugar level can go up. Elevated blood sugar levels for a long time can complicate our body systems and can damage our vital organs. So each and every organ of our body has a definite purpose. All are meant for a definite job or action.

"Life is a series of experience."

Every moment we are experiencing our life. We are planning every moment and little little habits often change our life. When we practice anything consistently and continuously it becomes habits in our life.If we practice happiness all the time, after sometime, it becomes a habit. The basic science for a better life is to keep ourselves always happy. Happiness is a choice and we need to be happy in any circumstance.If you can do something and can change the situation then it's OK and if you cannot change anything then also it's OK because it is not in your hand.So, in both the cases you are OK. If you can't change anything then it's OK but this often make life miserable for most of the people. We need to set priorities in our life. Our priorities must be defined with a clear deadline so that there is no chaos in our life. However, most of the time,we forget to define our priorities,we mess up our life by giving less importance to our important work. We need to feel the contentment in our life. Be content with what you have in life and ask the Universe to fulfill your other desire in life.

The purpose of humans on this earth is to balance the ecology with their intellect. We are born with a definite purpose and we need to do whatever we are meant to do.The purpose of our life is the most important discovery on this planet.

I remember clearly when one thought ignitedon 21st May,2005 and I was shaken. I was doing excellent in my professional carrier and was a content person. I am from a very humble background andstudied management with an ambition. I started my career a little late because I lost my six years after graduation in exploring different career options. I was searching for stability in my career and was unable to find it. Then again I started studying management to gain momentum in my career. I began my corporate carrier in 1998 and steppedonto the corporate ladder. I was very much determined that I will do well in my industry which I did and people recognized me. I switchedover to a few companies and changed my role,I went into training and development. I was a keen learner and read a lot about the industry. I took different technical trainings from different people and was very eager to learn the behavior pattern of the highly successful and happy people around me and I follow them very minutely. They are very well-organized people and a keen learner. It was an unbelievable experience to know people and their behavior patterns. I will never forget that day when I realized that all happy and successful people are different and their mindset is clearly different from normal people. I dreamed to be a happy and successful person from that day and I started reviewing people from different angles. I traveled a lot and observed different individual and their behavior patterns. I interviewed them,engagedin a conversation with them and gathered their personality traits. I was amazed that their perception ofhappiness and success is completely different. They made their destiny on their own. Maximum people drovefrom rags to riches in a systematic way and they always survived in adverse situations because they believe that anything is possible in life if we have theright mindset. They are very much determined about their decisions and failures. I was more excited to understand their routines. They are a go-getter and more disciplined. They don't stop after any setback. They don't give up after any temporary failure and are always keen to explore new possibilities in the adverse condition. They have learnt these skills from someone whom they follow and all these skills are learnable. I started following them and attended their lectures in different forums. I had a dream to be happy and successful in life. I have been studying mind for the lastfifteen years and enjoying this journey. I have learnt all the skills from different Teachers, Gurus, Masters and Mentors and have been applying them in my life. I experienced all these skills and am very much confident that these skills can change your life as well.I and my team always talk about these learnable skills in my Seminars and Workshops. Our Seminars and Workshops are fully experiential.I have seen all the successful and happy people are always grateful for each and everything in their life. They always adopt the forgive-and-forget formula and move forward. Their emotions are not stuck in any small event or circumstance.They always move forward without getting attached to anything. If failure comes, they just take a lesson and move forward.Duing my entrepreneur journey, I have used all these formulas to keep myself focused and firm. I am really happy and grateful to all of my Teachers, Gurus, Masters and Mentors for their unconditional contribution in my life. I could not have been an entrepreneur until and unless I trained my mind. I have struggled a lot but it was an adventure and rather I call it mad adventures. A journey of an entrepreneur is like a roller-coaster ride and you have to tie up the belt properly or else the chance of falling is inevitable. I had many ups and downs in this journey and I only used my Mindpower because I knew only mindpower can take me out of the situation. All adverse situations give me opportunities and I really observe it minutely. I transform the entire adverse situation into opportunities and come out of it.

Once our industrialist Mr.Ratan Tata said:

"UPS AND DOWNS IN LIFE ARE VERY IMPORTANT TO KEEP US GOING BECAUSE A STRAIGHT LINE EVEN IN AN ECG MEANS WE ARE NOT ALIVE."

This is a very strong statement and I always utter this statement in any adverse situation. I always believe that a person can choose happiness and misery. Nothing is static and everything is changing with every moment,from our cells in the body to the solar movement. We have to accept that success and failure are a part of our life.

Great scicntist Elbert Einsteinsaid that life is like a Cycle and we need to move on to prevent the fall. Success and failure are a part of the same cycle, we need to move on with these two. We are always broken down by any small failure and never recall that Thomas Edison failed for ten thousand times before his great invention of the electric bulb. We don't have the patience to even bear a small failure. Our motivation level is drops in case of any adversity and we put our self into stress. Stress in the mind cannot open up our intellect. Whenever our mind is calm and cool, our intellect awakes and we can think in different ways.

Every day,every moment things are changing and new things are evolving, so we need to update ourselves every moment. Acquiring knowledge is an art but experiencing that knowledge is Science. In my initial days, I thought that I knew about my capacity but didn't realize that my capacity is stretchable and I can expand it. My Gurus taught me that I can increase my knowledge slowly and gradually and it won't be possible if I want to do it in a day or two. I was not interested in increasing my knowledge because I had a limiting belief that I know enough for my job. I was job-oriented and didn't understand that there is an outer world where I can gain much more than I have. I was not exploring anything at that time and was content with my job and knowledge. I was inspired by the successful people around me and that was what made me curious to dig deepabout their life. So I started exploring the successful people and observed closely their habits and mental state. They are mentally very much stable and very much disciplined in their life. I interviewed them on different occasions and collected the data. Most of them are very much focused on their work and they know exactly what they want in life. They are very much systematic,they plan their work in advance and set their priorities. They know the difference between their urgent work and important work. All successful people I observed have a habit of writing every small thing in their notebook and review it on a regular basis. I was literally curious to know more about them and my journey began since then. I have been studying the mind and still learning. I was not good at academics and was not sure about my career. I was not much exposed to academics and career. During those days only doctors, engineers and lawyers were the best profession and beyond that, we never thought of anything. If we were not one among these three professionals, we were not considered successful in our life. There was no internet exposure and media exposure because the digital media was not developed. Information sharing was not very well established and we were dependent on print media. After the social media and digital revolution, the world has turned into a global village and we can access data from these sources. New courses have evolved and we can learn so many things from the online portal. Digital courses are available for different fields and all are easily accessible. We need to develop a tendency to learn as much as possible which can be developed only after gaining certain knowledge. We need to create a burning desire which is possible only when we have a big dream. I had a big dream and I started chasing my dream. A bigger dream can inspire us to take bigger action. We need to live with our dream. Taking action towards our dreamwill lead us to success. A dream without action is merely a wish and action without a dream will take us nowhere. I have experienced it myself. I was an average student in my academics and was not sure whether I can do something in life or not. I was inspired by many people and their struggle in life when I was searching for a job. Initially, I liked my job very muchbut got boredom after a few years. My mind often catapulted a question at me, 'What next?' I then again switched to a new job with a new role and enjoyed for a few years but again my mind asked the same question 'What next?' This 'What next' transported me to a completely new dimension and I started exploring mind because every time it was my mind that was the source of this question. I met different people on those days and studied about the mind and it's potential. I had a mental picture of mind and its true potential. I studied the human mind extensively and still studying to understand it fully. We have a different belief system and I have experienced it,for example, I had a belief that only doctors, engineers and lawyers can be successful in life. It was a myth because I broke this belief system,I worked on myself and my mind. I rewired my mind and set a goal that I will be successful and happy without these three. I changed my mental picture and ranked other professionsequivalent to these three. I wanted to be a happiness coach and share my happiness with the people around me. It was a very challenging task and I took this challenge positively. Determination can put you into action. It was not convincing for my family and I literally faced a hard time convincing them that there is a new world outside my job and I need to explore it. This was a risk but I was confident and my will power was immense. I pushed myself out of my comfort zone.It was like an uphill task during my initial days and I again went back to my comfort zone. I tried several times and adopted several methods to come out of my comfort zone and ultimately after a long struggle I am uncomfortable now. I made up my mind that my uncomfortable zone is my comfortable zone and I am very much comfortable in my uncomfortable zone. I was very scared of taking decisions and always had a fear of failure. Slowly and gradually I was convinced by the successful people that failure is the key to success. I always follow the rule of failure differently. So I took all the hard decisions in my lifewhile being full of confidence and accepted failure as a process of any success. I failed differently but not measurably. I was determined to do something new in my life and finally, I said goodbye to my corporate career. I quit my last assignment amicably and was released after six months because they did not want to lose me. Whatever studies I did were not possible until and unless I quit the job because I felt that if I want to do anything extraordinary then I have to be free from my corporate assignment. I won't be able to justify both the assignments at a time. If I am completely focused only then I can expect the outstanding outcome. I started exploring my masters during my corporate career and countered very few of them. I was convinced that they do things differently and they are very stable. I attended one hundred and twenty three workshops of different masters and took maximum lessonsfrom them. One thing was common in them which is consistence. All of them say one thing that regular practice of anything would become a habit after a few days. It depends on person to person, some take thirty days to make it a habit and some take ninety days.Once you are habituated then it would change your pattern. I took sixty-two days to make these practices my habit. Since then I do it regularly. If I miss out on something on a particular day then I feel that something is missing in my life. These practices are so powerful that it gives me unlimited energy and I am very much focused. I always coach people in my workshops about all these practices. I faced so many adverse situations in my career and life. I lost my mother in the year 2012 and I was shaken fully but because of these practices, I came out of that trauma. My mother was the only inspiration for me.

She was not educated much but she was really an extraordinary person. She kept her emotions aside and encouraged me to go out and do something visible to the society. I am happy and grateful to her for bringing me on this planet. When I was struggling to get a job, she supported me and she was very rigid. She said one thing,"Whatever wealth your father has, belongs to him,itsnot yours.You need to make your own identity and destiny." That time, I was not convinced by her thought but now I realize that she was absolutely right and outstanding. It was her dream and I made it my dream. I never thought that I could ever visit any new state apart from West Bengal but it was made possible because of her. She seemed to benot attached to me during my struggle but I knew she was always there and inspired me to establish myself. She used to say that make your own identity in this society and only knowledge and study can capacitate you to do that. I am really grateful to God for giving me a mother like her. I always follow successful people and their mental state. One thing is common in them which I have repeated several times that they are very stable and they enjoy the adverse adventure. I have had gone through the adverse situation many times and came out without any negative consequence. The formula I follow is very simple "Only the action with a specific measurable, attainable, reasonable and time-bound goal can take you to the top." It's very easy to say but difficult to practice. If we practice it regularly, it will make our path smooth and we can reach our destination very smoothly within a certain time. I always advise people to set a specific goal and take massive action and live with that goal until and unless it is achieved. In my workshops, I use all the tools, techniques and strategy which I learnt to monitor our progress in life. I do happiness programs for people above 14 years of age.

CHAPTER 4

Beautiful Human Body& Sound Health

The human body is the most complex machine in this Universe. There are trillions of cells in our body. Thousands of activities happen in our body every moment. Research says that our body the most complex instrument in this Universe. We are doing all our activities through our body organs. Our all organs have a different role in our body and any malfunction inour organ manifests with some symptoms. It gives an indication for any malfunction of our body organs. Our brain and mind control our body and it has a mechanism to send signals to our body to respond in a particular way.

Any malfunction in our body organs release enzymes and chemicals that flow in the bloodstream. Our body consists of 70% water and our thoughts impact our body badly. Japanese scientist Masaru Emoto did a research on water and it is very well documented. He experimented it in a lake. He asked monks to pray beside the lake,after a few hours, he took out some water and placed it under the microscope.He observed that the crystal formed was amazing and it was nicely shaped. He did the reverse and requested the monks to recite some negative prayers to the water.After a few hours he took out some water and placed it under the microscope.He observed that the crystal was formed badly. We can find out more about this research on the websites. So if our body consists of 70% water then we can make out that the negative thoughts can destroy our body easily. Thought impulse emits energy and it comes back to us as per the law of nature. So, if we send negative thoughts then negative things would come to our life. All the thoughts release chemicals and these chemicals can be measured by testing our blood. It gives us an indication about the organ that is affected and what is the level of malfunction. Our mind controls our body and when the mind is not stable then it gives an indication through our body. Almost 90% of our diseases are Psychosomatic in nature. Lucy Hay in her book "You Can Heal Your Life" explains the diseases and their cause. Our life is beautiful but because of our ignorance, we create problems in our life. We first suffer mentally and then it manifests in our body. Our brain and mind receive information from our five senses.They process the information and give the command to our body organs. We need to keep our mind and body fit to achieve our maximum potential. Three things are required to keep our life beautiful. Exercise, Meditation and Food.

Exercise keeps our body fit. Yoga, Aerobic and even simple walking would help in shaping up our body. Morning exercise is better to get good results. Breathing techniques and Meditation are the only food for the mind. If we are physically and mentally strong then we can accomplish our desire in a righteous way. We are the creator of our destiny and we can make it as per our choice. Nowadays, people have made life too complex. Life can be made easy by following certain rules. We are very much stressed up in little little things and create problems in our life. We need to be mentally fit. Every up and down teaches us a lesson. We are always down when there is anything wrong in our life but cannot understand that the circumstances, people and events would change slowly. We don't have the patience to wait till the good things come. We are dull and stressed up and this continuous stress leads to high blood pressure and blood sugar. We feel less energetic and develop anger in small small things. Research says that 1 minuteof anger pumps up cortisol (Stress Hormone) which remains in our body for 6 hours. Therefore, we need to be aware of our anger. Controlling anger is an art thatcan be achieved by Breathing techniques and Meditation. When our mind is stressed up and agitated then our intellect sleeps and when our mind is calm and cool then the intellect awakens. We engage in all sorts of wrong actions during our anger state and this action leads to great problems in the future. We need to be aware of such things and cool down our mind by taking a few deep breaths. We can enhance our productivity by doing only the breathing exercise. Meditation can do magic. It's really required to meditate at least 15 – 20 minutes a day. It's a great mind booster and it will help us to make the right decisions. Make a routine for meditation and try to do it ata particular time in a day. If meditation is irregular then the effect is less. So we need to prioritize meditation in our life. Our body is our source of energy and if the body is not fit then we cannot do what we want to do. Exercise, Meditation and Food; these are the three things thatwill create magic in our body, mind and soul. Meditation reduces the cortisol level in our body and reduces stress. Cortisol is the stress hormone and it creates problems in our body. Cortisol is a toxin and has to be flushed out of our body. We have different happy hormones like Oxytocin, Dopamine & Serotonin. All these hormones release in our body in different situations and it keeps our body and mind happy and healthy. Our body is our spiritual place and we need to keep it clean. We do not care for our body and abuses it every now and then. Our mind regulates our body and we need to keep both mind and body clean.

There is a say that "Health is Wealth". Most of us are running after wealth but we don't care about our health. Health is the most precious thing in our life and whatever we do for our health is less than what it requires. Our physical health and mental health arevery much related toeach other. Physical health depends upon our mental health and we are not aware of it. Good health means agood physical body and good mental health. To keep our health in good condition, we need to do physical exercise and need to take nutritious food. Mental health can be improved by doing Meditation and breathing exercises. In earlier days, people used a formula "Early to bed and Early to rise" and they were comparatively very much fit as compared to our generations. Their physical activities didn't require any exercise and they maintained their physical body very well. Nowadays physical exercise is minimal and sitting in thesame posture for long hoursis common. We need to develop some habits which can be developed by some practices.

If health is good then we can do whatever we want to do but we forget this and suffer because we abuse our body abruptly and don't give value to it. Food is the most essential to maintain our body. All the junk foods deregulate our glycemic index in our body and it triggers the blood glucose level in our body. But because of our lifestyle, we do consume junk foods every now and then.

CHAPTER 5

Imagination of Magnificent Self-Love&Be a Loving Soul

Most of us are not aware of the word 'Self-Love' or 'Self-Care'. Actually we always pay attention to our family, friends, relatives, colleagues and others but forget to pay attention to the lovely person inside us. We always deprive ourselves by avoiding a genius person within us. We always care for our surroundings including family, relatives, friends, and colleagues and don't love our self. We are the mirror image of our life. Whatever we are from inside, we reciprocate the same outside. We don't recognise our inner-self throughout our life and suffer. If we start taking care of our inner world then the outer world will automaticallychange. We are busy doing all the work for others and do not care about our soul. Self-introspection is the method for self-love. Inner journey is the only option to know us very well. We need to do inner engineering to manifest self-love. We need to nosedive deep down into our inner-self and see the beautiful world inside us. If our inner world is beautiful then the outer world has to be beautiful. We can take full control of our life if we love our inner-self. If we know our inner-self and care about it then the outer world will be of similar kind. Self-love and Self-care is possible if we stand in front of the mirror and look at our eyes for a long time. We can observe a beautiful person inside us waiting for appreciation, love and care. We never do that and take all the wrong information through our five senses and keep it within. We neglect our beautiful inner-self and absorb the outer world. If we know our true potential then we can realize that a beautiful soul is waiting for love and care. We always see flaws and insecurities in others and do not realize that our outer world is the mirror image of our inner world and what we see in others is happening inside us.

We can practice self-love habits by staying alone for some time every day. If we practice it every day, it will turn into a habit after sometime. If we really want to love and care our self then we need to take out time and do self-introspection. It will give us a feeling of our inner–self,we can look inside and feel the beautiful soul inside us. We always care for our surroundings and forget to care about our self. Mirror-practicecan make us feel that we are beautiful. Emotions can come out and we need to let go the emotions if theysurface during self-love because we have never see our self in this way. People have changed their life by only doing the mirror-practice. It is a long process to practice and very difficult to follow if we are not determined to change our self. Self-acceptance is self-love. If we accept our self as we are then the problem is solved. However, we usually look at the mirror and say that I am not good; I am not good looking, etc. But if we accept our self fully as we are then the problem is solved. In the beginning, it would be difficult to even stand in front of the mirror. "But Practice makes a man/woman perfect."To learn more about the process, you can walk in to our workshops as demonstrate it precisely in our workshops. When we know our inner-self then we are enlightened and in love. We need to spent some time alone with our self and immerse within self. Self love is most important than others because you can observe a beautiful person inside you and reciprocate the same to others. It means if you love yourself then you can love everybody. We need to remove the grudges stored in our mind and love our self. If you want to be enlightened from inside then you require self-love because self-love will enhance our self-image and it leads toa good mood and as I explained that our outer peace depends on our inner peace. Self-love is a process and we can initially feel awkward to love ourself. People who love their self can love others because our outer world is the exact mirror image of our inner world.Self-love is very important to our own self and it can recognise a good human being inside us.

We need to cultivate self-love. We are busy loving the outer world and fulfilling our near and dear's love. We often forget to make our self happy. We are happy for others but not happy with our self. Self-love and self-care is not selfishness. We think that if we love our self then we are selfish and people will call us selfish. But it's an art and if you follow the process of self-love then nobody can make out that you love yourself the most. We need to learn to love our self. If you practice in front of the mirror it makes the process of self-love easy.However, people don't even want to stand in front of the mirror for a long time as they think that the mirror is the only thing to see our look from outside. But we never tried to find out our inner-self in front of the mirror. We need to do self-talk and self-affirmation to love our self. Repetition of self-affirmation can reach our subconscious mind and helps us to love our self. We need to practice this self-love process everyday to make it a habit. If we follow it for minimum of 90 days then we can make it a habit.

Love is the second most vibration in this Universe. We forget to love and care about our self as we discussed that self-love and self-care are very important.As already stated our outer world is the mirror image of our inner world so if the inner world is in love then the outer world would automatically be in love. We love people conditionally and because of our interest we love others. Love should be spontaneous to everyone and people can feel our presence if we are in the vibrationof love. It has to be developed because the past conditioning restricts us from true love. In our childhood we wereconditioned thatpeople are bad, everybody is selfish, everybody loves because of their own interest, etc. Such negative statements are the factors that restrict love. If we radiate love without any condition and from the bottom of our heart then we can gain true power as we know that it can draw power from the Universe. Love is a fragrance and people can smell it very well. We do love our family members and surroundings but don't realize that whether it is out of compulsion or not. Our Heart Center is responsible for love and affection and if it is full of grudges then love would be artificial and it is not true love. We need to clean our Heart Center first and then love can manifest. We always take negative information from the Universe and absorb everything. We do not know the process to filter it out. This negative information gives us negative feelings and as our feelings come from the Heart Center, it blocks our Heart Center. If our Heart Center is blocked then we cannot feel love within our self. We need to first understand that we are really blessed to have this human life and only Love can bring us closer to everyone. If we love unconditionally then the Universe will bring more love in our life. It is the Universal law. We need to love our self first and observe that love comes to our life in many folds. Our mind givesthe signal to our heart after processing the information from our five senses and our heart is the centerof our emotion. If we feel sad then our whole body will work against our will. Our feelings come from the Heart Center and feelings create a vibration.If we feel love our inner-selfthen it brings more love into our life. Love comes from the heart centerand if we create all the grudgesin the heart centerthen love will not manifest. If you are in love with someone then it gives feelings in your heart centerand if that person comes in front of you then the heartbeat increases and feelings comefrom the heart centeronly. We can feel something happening inside our heart center,immediately our palpitation increases and we can feel enlightened if it is true love. Love is a feeling and if we spread love in society then society will reciprocate the same but the condition is that it should be unconditional. We always have grudges in our mind and it pierces our heart which gives us negative feelings and the negative feelings pump the Cortisol hormone in our body. Love can heal any wound which is deep-rooted. To clean our heart, we need to engage ourselves in forgive and forget practices. If we can clean our Heart then we can spread Love to all. If we send out love to the Universe then more love would come to us. As per the Universal law if we send out any vibration to the Universe then the same vibration would come to our life in many folds. We are conditioned in such a way that any work can be completed by anger which has negative consequences. Love can achieve anything without any condition. Love brings peace in our life. We need to learn how to increase our love vibration. We need to rewire our subconscious mind so that it can remove all the grudges from our past experience and eventuate inpositive progress in our life. We are the creator of our life and our life is dependent upon our feelings. Feeling is the most important thing to create vibrations. If we have negative feelings then we will create negative vibrations and if we have positive feelings then we will create positive vibrations. These vibrationsreside in our cellular level and we can feel it. Negative emotions ferry negative feelings in our cellular level and positive emotions trasport positive feelings in our body. Our body receives the signal from Amygdala in our brain and all our organs work as per the instruction of our mind. Love can solve any dispute and for that, we need to be in the same frequency with others. Love can be seen in any relationship but this relationship can be broken because of thlack of love. If we are neglected in our childhood then we search for love elsewhere and if somebody loves us then we reciprocate the same. Conditional love is temporary because it has some interest but unconditional love is permanent. Love can be temporary if it is one-sided because one person can feel love but the other is completely ignorant of it. One-sided love won't last for long. If it is from both sides then it can last for a longer period but condition applies. Love brings people closer. Love can be expressed in many ways and it depends on person to person. If somebody is madly in love with someone then it sometimes hurts them the most because the expectation is more out of that love and if the expectation is not fulfilled then it hurts.

True love can be seen by the len of feelings and feelings can come from our heart. If we are deprived oflove then we search badly to be loved by someone. Our subconscious mind can bring authentic people into our life. Falling in love feels like a vibration in our cellular level as our mind sends signals to our heart and the body reacts in that response. All good hormones like Oxytocin, Dopamine and Serotonin release in the body if you are in love and it shifts the mood of a person. These hormones changethe algorithm in our body and give us happy feelings. Love is a blessing from the Universe and we need to respect that. We ought to spread it every time. We can radiate our inner world to the outer world.

CHAPTER 6

Attitude of Gratitude

Gratitude is the highest vibration in this Universe. We always take everything for granted. We never appreciate what we have in life or what we have accomplished in our life.We think that everything is our birthright. We forget to thankothers for their kind help and support. We are not grateful forall the things we have in our life. We never show any gratefulness to people, nature and surroundings. What is the most essential thing for us to survive? AIR is the most important thing we require to survive. AIR is free for our whole life and we have not paid even a single penny for that. It is available in abundance in this Universe. We never feel grateful to the Universe for the AIR.We take it for granted that it is our birthright to get the AIR. There is abundance of everything in this Universe and we must be grateful for everything we have in our life. We need to create an abundance mentality.Our attitude towards gratitude should be very strong so that we can live our life with this gratitude mentality in everything we have in our life. However, we forget to harbour the gratitude mentality in our life. We are not happy and grateful for our achievement in life.We are always looking for the other things thatwe don't have in our life and feel sad. The first and foremost thing is to be grateful to the Universe for all the things we have then we can magnify our desire. Desire is the seed of any creation. We have to have a desire but at the same time whatever we have in life, we have to be grateful for that. We need to practice gratitude in every small thing in our life.When we wake up, we should first start the day with gratefulness and give thanks to God for that day because we are alive. So many people don't wake up the next day. It is true and we should thank the Universe for giving us the opportunity to serve another day. The Universe is so kind and it is like an ocean. If we draw a few buckets of water from the ocean every minute, we cannot empty the ocean, similarlyif we draw abundance from this Universe, we cannot make it empty. There is an abundance of everything in this Universe but we are unable to see it. To get the maximum water from the ocean we need to install a pipeline,similarly if we need to get maximum things from this Universe then we need to connect with it all the time. We are always busy with our chores and never bother to think in this way. If you want to make a fortune then the only way to get it is through gratitude because if you are there in that vibration, more of abundance comes to your life indifferent ways. We need to practice gratitude every moment to get maximum achievements. Universe has certain laws and it says whatever we send out to the Universe will come back to us. If we send gratitude to the Universe then more gratitude would come to our life. Every moment we can practice Gratitude by thankingfor everything we have in our life. Whatever small things we achieve in our life, we can be thankful for those. If somebody helps us in any small way, we can be thankful to the person.We must maintain an attitude for gratitude. All successful people practice it every moment in their life and they are blessed with more gratitude from the outer world. All happy people are full of gratitude in every moment of their life and they never complain aboutthe things they do not have. Desire can be created but it can't be at the cost of happiness.

More gratitude comes from the practice of gratitude and habits. Therefore, you must always affirm,"Thank you to every particle of this Universe." We seldom give any importance to the people around us who have helped usin any way and we take it for granted. We have to be grateful to every action that people take for us. When we feel gratitude within we will great and we will leave our ego behind. These feelings of gratitude enhance our happiness and we start respecting people who have helped us knowingly or unknowingly, directly or indirectly. It is the most powerful spiritual practices among all because it creates harmony in society and hatches the sense of belongingness. The only thing we need to understand is that only action is in our hand and the rest of the things are not. Everything is decided in this Universe and only the action can change our destiny. If we accept all the happenings wisely then we are happy. We should be grateful for all the works of the Universe and gratitude can expand our heart. We ought to be grateful to God for this amazing, wonderful, lovely, awesome, incredible life. We should be grateful for our parents for bringing us on this planet. We must be grateful to all of our organs for keeping us fit and fine. We should be grateful to Air, Water &Food for keeping us alive. We must be happy and grateful to all our family members for their blessings, teachings, love, help, support and kindness inour life. We should be grateful to all of our teachers, Gurus, Masters and Mentors for their unconditional blessings, teachings, love, help, support and kindness in our life. We ought to be happy and grateful to each and every particle in this Universe for their help, support, blessings, teachings, love and kindness to us.

Gratitude can expand our consciousness. It is the supreme vibration among alland we can expand our mind.

All happy people practice gratitude.It is in their DNA and they never forget to give thanks to every creature of this Universe.

The benefits of gratitude cannot be seen with an open eye but one can feel the difference while practicing it. People can see a difference in their behaviour which creates remarkable changes in their life.

People who practice gratitude in their day-to-day life can make a difference in other's life. If we feel that everything we are getting is not our creation and other's contribution then we can feel gratitude for others. Every act in this Universe depends upon many people and it is not only our creation. Like whatever crops we eat are not our creation, it is a creation of the farmers and so many people are involved to transport crops to our home. We only pay the price but if the farmer doesn't do the farming then we cannot get the crops. So we can be thankful to the chain of people who are actively involved in this process.

"Life is beautiful." We always think of our life. Life is awesome. We must always tell our self always that life is a gift from the Almighty. It's a great creation by the supreme power. Our life depends on us. We are the creator of our life. Our existence on this planet Earth is a blessing from the God. However, we always complicate our life by imitating others and feel dull. We are a unique creation of our creator and our life is completely different from the other creatures of this planet. We can create our life by using our intellect. The only difference between a human being and the other creature is that all human beings are equipped with intellect. To make our life full of wonder, we need to stop questioning about anything. Instead of questioning, we can wonder "How come". Life is filled with adventures. We need to romance with our life. We can achieve it by loving our life. Life is giving us everything.If a person is dead then instead of calling that person's name we call him or her a body. Body without life is like a perishable substance. We always think that this life is immortal. Our attachment in this life is very high because we do not realise that nothing belongs to us. We always show our abilities to everyone and wantthem to give us importance but if you are alone with your self then you can feel the company of a nice person. It's a precious gift by the Almighty to be taken care of very well.

CHAPTER 7

ReleaseEmotions through Forgiveness

Forgiveness is a great prayer!! Forgiveness is a great tool to clean our mind and heart. We are always emotionally hurt by thoughts, words and deeds. These words are very powerful and mightier than the sword. We always interact with people on a regular basis and we do not choose our words while talking to people;we communicate randomly. Forgiveness depends upon person to person. Wise people can forgive any act very easily because they don't keep it inside their mind.They clear the thoughts instantly. However, normal people always keep other's words or deeds in their mind and suffer a lot. Mental suffering is a self-created process and people carry it even till their last breath. They always hold the words and deeds in their mind and heart and live with them. Unhooking these words and deeds from their mind is an uphill task for them and they even don't want to search for a solution to unfasten the extra baggage. These grudges always block our mind for thoseparticular events, circumstances and people.Hence, we are unable to analyze or explore any new positive possibilities inside it. Forgiveness is a prayer that removes all the old thoughts, words and deeds over a period of time. It takes even more time if it is deep-rooted. We need to forgive people, not the act. If someone does something wrong to us then we need to forgive that person and take action about the act. In this process, we can release our self from the emotion. All successful people are very strong in forgiving other's thoughts, words and deeds very often. They forgive and go forward. "FORGIVE AND GO FORWARD" is the best way to move without baggage. Normal people hold it for a long time and search for an opportunity to retaliate. It's the most dangerous thing to hold on to for a long time and retaliate. Holding anything in our mind and heart gives us stress and whenever we encounter that event or circumstances then we are shaken. Wise people know it that "NOTHING IS PERMANENT". People hold these thoughts, words or deeds for a long time but do not recognise that the otherperson has already forgotten the event. If these people come to our life again with some opportunity, we just ignore them and lose that opportunity. It is very important to forgive people then and there and don't carry any extra luggage in your mind. Extra luggage occupies space in your mind and will not be removed until and unless you intend to remove it permanently. Forgiveness is an act for our wellbeing and it has nothing to do with others. It's an internal conflict and to resolve this conflict we need to be proactive and take all possible steps to get rid of this conflict. It's a great conflict in our mind and body and it will lead to more conflicts in asimilar situation. Similar events circumstances or people can come to your life frequently and you might have blocked your mind from any opportunity or possibilities from them in the future. We need to be wise on this front and move forward. Free flowing water is better than stagnate water in terms of quality,so we need to move forward for a better understanding rather than stagnate at one place with limited opportunities. Life moves on and we experience new things every moment. However, if we are stuck with all these baggage then we cannot explore our future because the mind is always occupied with the garbage. If we practice forgiveness on a daily basis then we are decluttering our mind on a daily basis. If we don'tclean our floor on a daily basis then the dust particleswill accumulate on the floor and it takes more time to clean. If we sweep everyday then the floor could be cleanedquite easily.Whereas, if we clean the floor once in a month then we have to work hard to remove the stains. Similarly, if we clean our mind on a regular basis then the dust in our mind can be cleaned easily. In every relationship forgiveness is the only tool to keep that relationship moving forward. It has been observed that people are stuck in these thoughts, words and deeds for a long time and they always resist to talk to the person who hurt them in the past. Always forgive others and move on. We sometimes abuse knowingly or unknowingly to our dear ones and forget to ask for forgiveness.This leads to conflicts and pain to the other person. Forgivenessis a great act and the person who is very strong can only forgive others. It's a sign of a strong person. Forgiveness is not the cup of tea of a weak person. Weak people hold the thoughts, words or deeds for a long time and lose their true potential by recalling thosewords or thoughts or deeds again and again. It's very hard to forgive others because we are conditioned to carry grudges for a long time. We have gathered information from our senses and look around them. We experience all these conflicts between people,we condition our self that these conflicts cannot be resolved and hold these for a long time. We take sympathy from others and enjoy our sadness as people give importance to a sad person. We attract people by using our sadness and gain sympathy. But sympathy cannot last for a long and if your tendency is to live with sadness then after sometimes people will not even sympathise with you because you are always in that state of mind. Forgiveness is a mental state and people are conditioned with their past experience to hold words or deeds in their mind. They think that if they forgive others then theyare going to be weak. It's a wrong conditioning that people who forgive arevery weak. Instead, it's a sign of boldness. If we forgive people, circumstances and events on a regular basis then we can forget it after sometimes and start a new chapter with a new thought. There are instances we feel hard to forgive because it is so deep-rooted. We need to practice forgiveness for a long time to remove those emotions. Sometimes we feel that we are not at fault and the other person doesn't say sorry at all then how can I forgive him or her? It's common for all of us. We need to acknowledge the fault from the other person's perspective and then forgive. However, it does not happen as the other person might think that it is not his or her fault because he or she saw the event from a different angle or perspective. Everybody is unique and their intelligence is also unique. So, it's very difficult for everyone to work in sync with your way,if they do not work in your way then conflict arises and we are unable to find out their logic and solutions. I have highlighted that we don't need to forgive the act but we must forgive the person. We sometimes see from the lens of the other person's actand don't see other's feelings because it is not seen easily. We sometimes hurt other's feeling knowingly or unknowingly but are unable to recognise the feelings. Sometimes we feel bad because someone hurt our feelings. In all such situation, we need to do the forgiveness prayer everyday for our self, not for others. Forgiveness will certainly remove the feelings and repair our mind and heart. God has given emotions to human beings and emotions is what separate us from the animals. We have to let go these feelings through forgiveness. Physical hurt is less expensive than emotional hurt. Physical hurt can be forgotten but the emotional pain during that time can't be forgotten easily. We need to GIVE AND ASK for forgiveness so that we can clean all the clutters stored in our mind. Actually, forgiveness is the act of removing emotional hurts. If someone hurts your emotion immensely, then it is very important to forgive him or her on a regular basis until it gets flushed out of your mind and heart.

CHAPTER 8

Result of a True Relationship

Harvard University has established a fact after an extensive study on relationship which was concluded recently and they have established the fact that the only key to great health and success is relationship. They have studied extensively and did research on relationship and came to the conclusion that if a person can maintain the proper relationship then he or she can achieve anything in their life. Relationship is the only vital thing in our journey of life. We actually fail to establish relationship very often. The human mind is always stuck and avoidsstepping in a new relationship because of past conditioning. Human mind conditioning is like People are Selfish, People want their work to be done with a wrong intention, People are jealous, People will not support me, People are cunning, People are not helpful, etc. We always restrict our self in our mind. It has been established that success is created twice first in our mind and the second in our physical world. Human mind is always preoccupied with past thoughts and conditioning and never tries to explore anything outside until one learns to rewire his or her mind. Trust deficit is the main reason for any relationship breakup. Relationship can either make you or break you. Relationships with the family members are vital to accelerate your highest potential and if we fail to establish that then life can be miserable. It is our mind thathas to clean all the old garbage to maintain a healthy and fruitful relationship. We need to forgive and forgetpast events or circumstances to establish a good relationship. It happens at our workplace wherein we sometimes get stuck at one issue,we are not able tomove forward and explore any new things. Our mind churns the same events or circumstances every moment and we are unable to come out of it. Any event which we think is wrong can be right for others. We have to be wise enough to see in a holistic way. We do not foresee the future because we are stuck in our past and exploiting our present. Relationship plays a key role in our life every moment. We sometimes think that there is no future in a particular relationship because our mind is stuck and we do not even look at it because our eyes are focused on the issues, not on the solutions. How can a person say that there is no future in a relationship? A successful and wise person knows how to re-establish a fruitful relationship when the relationship is on the verge of breakup. Our EGO is the culprit in establishing relationships because EGO does not allow us to think in another person's way. EGO is stuck in between and the question surfaces that why should I accept other's opinion. EGO kills us badly but we don't understand it,we keep on applying our own logic and spoiling the relationship. If sometimes we feel that this relationship won't last long then we need to part way amicably so that if we realise later .that it was our fault then we can go back and re-establish that relationship. Relationship with your spouse is the only relationship based on trust. If there is a trust deficit then it cannot go inthelong run. Most of the time our mind is preoccupied and doesn't listen to other's voice. Our subconscious mind can repair such relationship by reprogramming. Our subconscious programming can help us maintain a happy and healthy relationship. People say "look" does matter in any relationship but it's not the case. It's the trust which matters the most to carry a relationship. Before establishing any relationship we need to develop a rapport and gradually weneed to understand each other before making any commitment in that relationship. Our relationship doesn't last because of our impulsive decision that we take without understanding each other's likes and dislikes. Actually, our mind and thought frequency should match with the opposite person because energy transmission is required to establish a prosperous and healthy relationship. We all are connected in this Universe but we are disconnected internally because our receiver is weak and has a certain limitation. We need to re-establish the connection. As I stated earlier that our mind is a neurotransmitter and we send our thoughts to the Universe with a certain frequency.We use the similar frequency when we catch from the Universe. We are always stuck in small matters and don't allow our self to leave it aside and move forward. These small things are stuck in our subconscious mind and that doesn't allow us to maintain a relationship. In our workplace, we always negotiate with our relationship and carry on but do not try to explore that relationship. Relationship issues lead to health problems in our life and hence,we increase the Cortisol level in the blood which is a stress hormone. It increases the blood pressure and blood sugar level in our body. One minute's anger can pump Cortisol in our body and stay for SIX hours. We need to rewire our subconscious mind for our relationship. Relationship issue is the major issue in this decade and the productivity decreases because of this. A true relationship can make wonders. Long-distance relationship cannot last for a long time because emotional bonding is missing. Long-distance relationship is to just carry on without any strong emotional bonding. If we have a healthy relationship then we can feel it whenever that person is around,we are always happy when he is within our reach. Relationship is a feelingthat our mind can sense and send a signal to our heart. Relationship is attached to our emotion.

Keys for a healthy relationship:

1) Trustworthy

2) Lovable

3) Good understanding

4) Egoless

5) Truthfulness.

The human mind is very well designed by the creator. As we accepted anything in our childhood, it is stored in the hard disk. We absorb all the information from our five senses which are stored in our subconscious mind and carry it till our last breath. We need to reprogram it for our good, healthy and happy relationship.

Marriage relationship depends on the programming in our mind. Our subconscious mind is the only source to improve the quality of our married life. Command to our subconscious mind is very much vital and we need to activate it for any marriage relationship. Marriage can be very smooth if we understand our subconscious mind. Any relationship in our life depends on our subconscious programming. If we program our subconscious mind in a positive way then our marriage would be very much successful. A happy and healthy relationship can make people grow in their life. If we program our subconscious with positive affirmation on marriage then it will manifest. Anyone can start thisprogramming even well before marriage. It can be a positive affirmation on a marriage relationship. Infinite intelligence in our subconscious mind can make it happen sooner or later but the condition is that we need to have 100% faith and belief that it is going to happen. The secret of all the healthy and happy marriage relationships dependson thisprincipal. People are not aware of these secrets and hencc, their relationship suffers badly.

We need to understand why few people are successful and happy in their life. To understand the psychology behind success and happiness, we need to understand fourcharacteristics which we call QUOTIENT. The four quotients are:

1) Intelligent Quotient

2) Emotional Quotient

3) Spiritual Quotient

4) Social Quotient

Are all intelligent people successful? Not necessarily! Less intelligent people can be more successful than intelligent people. Research saysthat people who are emotionally strong can be more successful always because EQ(Emotional Quotient) is more powerful than IQ(Intelligent Quotient) and SQ(Spiritual Quotient) is the most powerful. We always observe a person is less intelligent and very well successful. Research says that success depends upon EQ and if a person's EQ is strong then the success rate is very high. The quotient ratio of success is 10% IQ and 90% EQ. We are always running after IQ and don't consider EQ at all and that's why it is being observed that highly intelligent people struggle to get success in their life. We need to see the EQ level for success. People who are emotionally very strong can achieve a great height in their career with less efforts. The spiritual quotient is more important because we need to understand our self very well. Self-introspection is the key to understand one's self. We need to understand ourselves in depth. To understand our own self, we need to take an inward journey by relaxing our mind and stay within self. We can understand our Subconscious mind and its power. We have to increase our own power through spiritual practices.

CHAPTER 9

Effects of Blessings

Blessing is an important part of our life. Blessings attract more blessings. We forget to acknowledge our blessings in life. We don't enjoy the present moment,we think about the past and are always worried about the future. We are not at all content,weare always unhappy about the present situation and we do not count our blessings. Let me explain it here. What is the most essential thing to live our life?As stated earlier, the first and foremost thing is AIR. Without air we cannot survive for a minute. But we never acknowledge it and think that it is our birthright. Next is water, without water we cannot survive for more than 3 days and we think that it is our birthright. Third is food. We are blessed with free Air and water in our life. Do we ever acknowledge that? Never!! We are unhappy because of the things we do not have. It isthe tendency of our mind to crave for the things which we do not have.Blessings are very important in our life. We are really blessed that we born as a human. We can always feel blessed as we are alive right now. When we wake up in the morning we feel that we have onc day more to live and it's a divine blessing. We need to always acknowledge our blessings and as I explained earlier that whatever we send out, it will come back in many folds. If we always say that we are blessed then more blessings arebound to come in terms of different things in our life. We can always be grateful forwhat we have in life and feel that we are blessed foreverything in life. I personally feel that I am really blessed for everything in my life and believe me I always get more than what I ask from the Universe. One of the most important things in our life are happiness and we always search for happiness on the outside but never look inside. If we feel blessed in life then happiness will come automatically. Our good health is a great blessing toour life. We are fit and fine, so we are really blessed. We need to count our blessings all the time in our life and we can see that there are so many blessings we have in our life. If you feel that you are blessed then the self-confidence will grow up in your life. You can feel it when you see people do not have what you have.If somebody doesn't have legs then we can feel that we are blessed with legs. If we see people sleeping on the roadside then we can feel that we are blessed with a home. If somebody does not have a car then we can feel that we are blessed with a car. So, there are numerous blessings in our life but we do not count them. Every small blessing needs appreciation.

We can see people have problems in relationship and are suffering badly, at the same time we feel that we are blessed with a lovely relationship. I always practice this exercise and feel that I am flooded with more blessings in my life. It is indeed a habit and we need to develop it over a period of time. Whatever works we perform in life just feel that you are blessed for that and do with full dedication and integrity. Actually, blessing can rewire our mind and keep negativity at bay. Our potential would be increased and the work would be half done when we feel we are blessed for everything in life.

CHAPTER 10

Develop a Money-Mindset

"***Money is energy***". Money-mindset depends on our childhood programming. Between 3 – 8 years of age, all the programming in different areas takes place and our belief system is conditioned that way. We always heard from our surrounding that "Money is the root of all Evils", Rich people are bad, Money won't grow on the trees, hard work is required to earn money, Rich people are corrupt, etc. These beliefs are conditioned in our mind and the results in our money area dependon our beliefs. Our life is the results of our thoughts. We carry this belief system till the last day of our life and act accordingly. Money area is an essential area of our life. We need to change our belief system. All rich people have a different belief system for money and they always attract money. Money cannot be destroyed. It can change hands but won't be destroyed. As per research, 1% of people in this universe hold 96% of the wealth. We see rich people become richer and poor people become poorer. Poor people put in their hard work but still, they are poor. Actually, the universal law is different and we are not aware ofthe law. Our subconscious mind is fully conditioned by our surroundings and we believe in that all the time. We can reprogram our subconscious mind to change the belief system and get better results in the money area. Repeated self-affirmation and self-talk can recondition our mind and belief system. We need to develop the money mindset so that we can get maximum results. If we condition our mind then we can achieve our desired goal. Visualization is a process where we can enhance the possibilities as our subconscious mind cannot recognise real events happening or visualization happening. If we visualize we can actualize. Our belief system won't allow us to visualize because our old belief system stops us from doing that. We need to dive deep down in our subconscious mind and do this process of conditioning. We need to change our belief system,we ought to reprogram our mind and act like a rich person. Inthe beginning, it will not allow us to believe it but during this repeated process, our mind can change and our subconscious mind can believe that it's true. Self-talk or affirmation is a very powerful tool to recondition our mind but at the same time it is difficult to develop trust in the same.Therefore,people leave it in between and the results do not come as per the expectation. All rich people are conditioned from childhood and if they fail to achieve the amount of money they desire,the failure will not last forever,they can bounce back very easily. In any adverse condition, if rich people lose some money they can bounce back within a very littleamount of time. Where is the problem? It's the problem in our childhood conditioning. We conduct the "Millionaire Mind Unlimited" workshop to change the belief system and achieve the millionaire mindset.

CHAPTER 11

Life without Vision, Goal and Action

Successful people are always visionaries,they have their vision with conviction and confidence. Their actions are always vision-oriented and they know what they need in life. I have interviewed several happy and successful people,as per them happiness is a choice and they always pretend themselves to be happy in any situation. Happiness is a very strong vibration,it aligns our neurological settings and drives us to take action with a positive mindset. If we are happy then success would touch our life. Our happy hormones like Endorphin, Oxytocin, Dopamine and Serotonin are releasedon different occasions when we are happy and these hormones help us to act differently to achieve the set goal. When you are clear, you tune into the exact vibration. There are different vision exercises to make it a reality. It doesn't matter whether your vision is very high or very low. If we always follow our vision then we can achieve any of our set goals very fast. Vision exercise isvery powerful and changes our mind. Actually, we give command to our subconscious mind during vision exercise and our subconscious mind attracts people, circumstances and events to our life to accomplish the vision.

"Limitations live only in our minds. But if we use our imaginations, our possibilities become limitless."

– Jamie Paolinetti

The Vision Exercise:

Clarify your Vision in all the Seven Areas of your life to configure the Inner GPS System:

1) Health/Appearance
2) Relationship
3) Financial
4) Career
5) Free time/Family time/Recreation
6) Personal(Including learning)
7) Community

We can share our vision for maximum Impact. Our vision affirmations can bring us back to the right track.

1) Health:

Health is the most important asset of our life.

Our statement about Health:

- I am healthy. All of my organs are in harmony and aligned with each other.
- My body is very powerful and all of my body parts are working day and night to keep me fit and fine.
- Every cell in my body vibrates with energy and health.
- I love my body. My body is very smart and gives me a signal for any new information.
- My, Heart, Lungs, Liver, Gall bladder, Intestine, Pancreas and Kidneys are working every moment to keep myself healthy and alive.

2) Relationship:

Relationship is one of the most important parts in our happy living. Research says that relationship is the only parameter in our life which can decide our happiness. 80% of our happiness depends upon the relationship we maintain in our life. Relationship is responsible for our personal and professional achievements. It is a very very important factor forour accomplishment.

Our Statement about Relationship:

- My relationship with each and everyone is awesome.
- I maintain a healthy relationship with each and every individual.
- I am having a great relationship with each and every creature of this planet earth.
- My relationship with my family is excellent and my family members reciprocate the same.
- My relationships with all of my professional colleagues are excellent and they also maintain the same.
- I maintain a loving relationship with my social circle and they return me the same.

3) Financial:

Finance is important to live our life with contentment. Our financial health depends upon our programming during the childhood. If our belief is wrong about money then we cannot hold a healthy financial life for a long time. Our belief system is responsible for our finance in life. If our beliefs are like, rich men are not honest; money cannot grow on trees, all rich people are bad, rich people are arrogant, earning money is very hard, etc.,these programmings are permanently stored in our subconscious mind and we act like that. We do not want to be rich because Rich people are bad. We do not ask for money because money cannot grow ontrees. If we are not arrogant andwhen we are rich even then we would not be arrogant. Money and finance are the tools for our successful living.

Our statement aboutFinance:

- My financial health is very strong. I am rich.
- I earn money easily and effortlessly.
- Money comes to my life consistently and on a continuous basis.
- Money loves me.
- Money is my friend.

4) Career:

We are very much career-oriented and always have concerns about our career and growth in life. We are not content at all and we search for options. There are countless career options in front of us and we switch over very frequently because we do not identify our purpose and we are not very happy with our existing career. We need to find our purpose and choose our career options according to that. If we are very happy with our work and enjoying it then we can think that we are on the purpose of our life.

Our statement about the career:

- My career is at its peak.
- I am enjoying every work in my career.
- I am a career focused and career-oriented person.
- I can choose a new career option easily and effortlessly.
- I am blessed with my lovely career.

5) Free time/Family time/Recreation:

We work like a machine and we forget to give our self free time. We are always in the rat race and running here and there without a break. We are unable to take out free time for our self, our family and any recreation. All the successful people whom I interviewed have confirmed that their time is very much planned and they keep free time for themvels, their family and recreation. They believe that these three spaces can rejuvenate them and take their life to the next level. As per them, the human mind needs some sort of recreation and if we can nurture our inner child then we can free our mind from all clutters.

Our statement about the Free time/Family time/ Recreation:

- I enjoy my free time alone with the happiest and successful person on this planet.

- I spend my free time with Nature.
- My enjoyment starts with my family gettogether.
- Playing and listening to music always enlighten me and gives soothing effects to my mind and body.

6) Personal:

All the happy and successful people separate their personal life from their professional life. They do not carry their professional work to their home and vice versa. They detached themselves from the outer world and focus on their family and recreation. They are a very good learner and they are always in learning mode. Reading books is ahabit for most of them. Learning is their personal hobby and they spend most of their free time reading books and in recreation.

Our statement about Personal Life:

- I enjoy my personal time with myself.
- Family time is being kept during personal time.
- Leaning is my hobby and I learn through reading books.
- Spending personal time with myself is thehappiest moment for me.

7) Community/Social:

Due to over commitment at workplace and family, we always forget our social life and the community. Social life is very very important to serve the society. Human being is born to do something for the society and community. Social responsibility gives us power and recognition. We are recognised by our work towards the society. All the happy and successful people always serve the society in a different way. Social recognition and getting help from the society is required for a person to live his or her life. Relationship development is a must for our social development.

Our statement about Community/Social Life:

- I serve the community and take responsibility to develop a healthy relationship.
- I admire and respect people all the time.
- Social recognition gives me happiness and joy.
- I involve in social work and enjoy the job.
- I love my society and community for their contribution to my life.

Goal Setting

For converting Vision into Reality, we need to set GOALS, which are measurable and Time-bound.When setting Goals, make sure:

1) Goals need to be balanced

2) Goals need to be SMART

3) Goals must have a Purpose (of making a difference to self and others). Goals should take care of the environment.

Goal Balancing:

Health / Appearance – Weight, fitness, looks, aging, food habits

Relationships – bringing aliveness, building new relations, kindof people you want to attract into your life

Financial – Income, Savings, Home, Car, Material things

Career – Position,Compensation,Customers, Colleagues

Balancing your goals across all aspects of your life.

Free Time / Family Time – spending 1-2-1 time, social events, travel, fun/leisure activities

Community – Giving back (time/money), Contribution, making a difference in people's lives, community activities, Spiritual Goals

Personal (including learning goals) – hobbies, learning goals, marathon, travel, spiritual journey

SMART Goals for 100% Clarity, we must set SMART Goals...

S – Specific (Clarity)

M – Measurable (Trackable)

A – Attainable (Your Beliefs)

R – Realistic (As per nature)

T – Time-bound

Ensure clear commands to the Genie who is sitting inside us.

Goal Setting: Some Tips for Goal Setting...

Have one Goal which can give a QUANTUM LEAP to your professional or personal life. This Is your Breakthrough Goal.

Also, make your Bucket List... 101 Goals you want to achieve before you die.

Always write your Goals with your hand because handwritten goals are always registered in your mind

Connect with your Goals three times a day and visualize all the time that it is happening in front of you.

Goal Setting Examples:

Examples of SMART Goals

Health Goals - I will exercise 4 times a week for 30 minutes starting from 1st March 2020 at 5 am in the morning.

Relationship Goals - I will spend at least 30 minutes with my family members every day starting from Saturday, 14thMarch,2020.

Study Goals - I want to score 95% in my board exams in March2020.

Career Goals - I want to become the Vice President of my company by 1stJune 2020

Financial Goals - I want my monthly income to be Rs. 2 lakhs starting from 1st April,2021.

Hobbies - I want to join a guitar class by 1st September 2021

Things you want - I want to live in a 4 bedroom house at Jorbagh, New Delhifrom 1st October 2022

Any other dream - I want to travel around the world with my family starting from 1stJuly 2023.

Unleash the Power of Goal Setting. "How" Do I Achieve My Goals?

We need to prepare some tools to stay FOCUSSED on our GOALS

If you are focused then you can realize the power of focus.

Mind Tools - Prepare the following tools:

- Prepare a Vision Board for your long term goal and put it in front of your bed so that you can visualize all those long term goals frequently.
- Every night before going to bed just go through the Goal Affirmation workbook and visualize.

Two other invaluable tools:

- You can always carry a Small Ideas Bookin which you write down all the ideas that pop up during the day. These ideas can be analyzed regularly and explored for the possibilities.
- Daily writing in a Gratitude Journal is a must. If you are grateful for small things then just pen down in the gratitude journal. It will bring more opportunities.
- At the end of the day just write all the achievements of the day in the Victory Log Book on a regular basis and check weekly how much did you accomplish.

Connecting with the Genie

Three ways to connect:

- We need to connect with our subconscious mind everyday, at least twice, by relaxing our mind.

- Long Relaxation technique.

Technique 1: Visualization and Guidelines for Visualization

- Must be done in Relaxation State. You need to visualize the things happenings right in front of you.
- Our Subconscious mind loves movies, so make sure you need to visualize that the movie is running inside your mind right now. Visualizing the pictures clearly in front of you can make it possible.
- Visualize with feelings of complete faith that the goal has happened and you are very happy after achieving the goal.

  See What You Want, Get What You See!

Technique 2: Affirmations

What is an Affirmation?

Every thought you think and every word you say is an Affirmation.

Thoughts and Words mixed with emotion create Vibrations, which create our life realities.

What is "Practicing Affirmations"?

"Practicing Affirmations" means saying out statements (with passion and feelings):

- Which assume that your Goal has already been achieved OR
- Which depict the way you would like to see yourself or the way you would like to experience your Life

Affirmations (Technique)

Two types of Affirmations

1) ***Goal Specific Affirmations*** – Statements thatconfirm your Goal is already achieved.
   - I am so happy and grateful that my monthly income is now Rs. 2 lakhs.
   - I am celebrating for feeling light and alive in my perfect body weight of 76 kgs.
   - I am feeling so proud and happy for having invented a new technology that will make a huge difference to my customers.
   - I am excitedly watching orders pour in over the internet for my new products.
   - I am feeling so proud to be graduating in the top of my class with honors.
   - I am happily stepping through the door of my brand new dream home.

Dealing with obstacles in the goal-achievement process

- Two types of Roadblocks: Internal and External Roadblocks. Our internal roadblocks are imposed by our belief system and the external roadblocks are due to Govt. Policies, Rules, Regulation and Statutory, etc.
- Negative Vibrations, Negative Thoughts, Negative Emotions, Limiting Beliefs,Low Vibrations, Past Negative Experience, past hurt, guilt, sadness, Self Image Issues, Body Pain, Unwell.
- Limiting Beliefs, Self-limiting belief and self-imposed limitation.
- Our Beliefs drive our entire life and these beliefs are the programming in our childhood.
- A thought which we assume to be true is a Belief.
- Beliefs can be of two types – empowering and disempowering.
- Beliefs are formed by Socio-Economic – Educational - Religious conditioning.
- Beliefs are the Operating System thatdrive everything we do.
- Our Core Beliefs are formed before the age of 8 years. 3 - 8 years of age is very crucial for a child because

in this period all the programs are installed. Before 3 years of age, a child's mind is like an empty hard disk.

"Whatever a human mind can conceive and believe, it can achieve."

-Napolean Hill

- Limiting beliefs are a part of our operating system. It can be redesigned by installing a new program and a new operating system.
- A Limiting Belief is one that holds us back fromachieving our Goals. We need to find out our old beliefs and rewrite them with a new positive belief system. It takes a long time to root out the old belief system and install a new positive belief system.
- Limiting beliefs are formed due to conditioning or past experiences. Since our childhood, we listen to all these old beliefs and hence these got stored permanently in our subconscious mind. Whenever we want to do a new thing,this belief will disallow it to happen.
- There are two types of limiting beliefs – conscious self-defeating beliefs and sub-conscious self-defeating beliefs.
- These programs run automatically without our knowledge because we have stored these programs

since our childhood and have never rewritten those with a new program.

- Beliefs play a major role in Goal Achievement. If our belief is negative then we cannot achieve our goals even after pouring in all the hard work because our subconscious is very powerful and it will work against those beliefs.

Affirmations (Technique)

2) ***General Positive Affirmations*** – Simply affirm your positive beliefs about yourself and your life.

- My life is abundant in every way.
- I am successful in all that I do.
- I create miracles in my life.
- I easily find solutions to any problems.
- My life is filled with love and beauty.
- I am divinely guided and protected.
- I am attracting joy into my life.
- I am loved.
- I can do anything.
- I make a difference inthis world.

Remember that the affirmations are like SEEDS. They look like a LIE but they have the potential to convert into REALITY. We need to releasc thebrakes to move on.

Divine planning:After programming the genie, it will do divine planning and attract opportunities, people, events, ideas, and resources towards us. We need to identify the opportunities.

Subconscious mind will inspire you to take action. It will communicate back through intuition,dreams,hunches, & Flashes.

Take action: Taking massive action is a must. Only action can give the right direction. We must then keep our antennae **ON** at all times i.e. be alert. Capture Ideas and Inspiration received from the Genie. Notice People coming into your life, invitation to Events and Opportunities coming to you.

Take OBVIOUS and INSPIRED Action. Keep taking ACTION.

Don't get stuck for the right time, right place, etc. Start taking small small actions.The right time will never come. First take action and then make it right.

Follow the Principles of ASK, ASK, ASK and Reject the Rejection. We are always hesitant to ask anything from anybody. Always ASK, ASK, and ASK. Repetitive asking can make others think. Rejection can come for several times but never stop asking. After repetitive rejections, one can still expect if he has a strong belief in himself.

Ready, Fire, Aim: Actually, if we fire first and then aim then it is very easy to accomplish our goal because we can experience more. Failure can keep us closer to our success.

Be **patient and expect** the results at any time (be in expectancy mode). Keep on PERSISTING.

If actions are not giving results, Seek feedback (Internal and External). Internal feedback can be taken from our subconscious mind and external feedback can be taken from all the external resources.We can use E + R = O formula (Events + Responses = Outcome) to understand our response and the outcome.

Persist until you SUCCEED. If Failures show up, learn and Move forward. Use all the TOOLS to stay on TRACK. Persistence is the key to stay on track. Have faith in yourself and make consistent efforts. One idea can give you success if you have faith and belief on that idea. Massive action takers fall and stand up very fast and they are unstoppable because they are inspired by their actions.

The key is to NEVER EVER GIVE UP... KEEP FAITH that your Goal will happen. YOU WILL HAVE TO PASS THE FINAL TEST.

Achieve Results: Celebrate Success to bring happiness in our life. Even a small achievement is a great inspiration for us to take massive action. We always forget to celebrate small achievements in our life and wait for the big achievement which takes a long time. Celebration of small achievement can boost up our energy and we put consistent and persistent efforts for the big achievements. If we don't celebrate our small achievement then the self-motivation for the big tasks would be very less.

Completion

NEVER EVER GIVE UP ATTITUDE!! We can learn it from the famous inventor Thomas.A.Edison. He failed 10000 times and he had developed a never-ever-give-up attitude. We can adopt this attitude by counting the failures of all the famous people that they faced in their life. Failure or defeat is temporary and we can get feedback aboutour work through failure and defeat. If you want to be Unstoppable then you need to adopt the never-ever-give-up attitude.

RAISING VIBRATIONS!! Vibrations can be raised by positive people. Always surround yourself with positive people. Raising your vibrations can increase productivity. Energy can be evolved and we can channelize this energy in a positive way. Rising vibration can boost up efficiency and effectiveness of our work and can help us in accomplishing our goal in a very simple way.

Living in alignment with the Universe. It is being observed that if we are aligned with the Universe and followNature then we can draw all good things in our life. Universe is giving us everything without even being asked. Air and water are the two most important things for a living being. There is an abundance of Air and water in this Universe. If we are fully aligned with the Universe then we can avail everything from it. We have to be happy and grateful to the Universe foreverything in our life.The more we are grateful the more we can receive from it.

Eat *satvik* food:

The foods which increase life, purity, strength, health, joy and cheerfulness

- Brings purity and calmness to the mind
- Soothing and nourishing to the body
- Raising Your Vibrations

Adopt a forgive-and-forget attitude. It is very much required for our mind to drop the unwanted luggage. We always carry thoughts, words and deeds and we don't want to forgive people for their wrong words and deeds towards us. We carry it for a long time and our mind is occupied with that. If we practice a simple forgiveness prayer then we can recalibrate our mind and can find our true self. It is our nature to hold any word or deeds for a long time. We can practice the forgiveness prayer anytime when we feel the requirement and it is very effective if we practice it immediately after the wrong things happen with us. We can forgive people instantly and relieve us from that pain. We don't want to forgive the act but we can forgive the people. If he or she comes to our life next time then we won't feel any wrong vibration inside us.

Regularly observe silence. Silence is agreat tool for our mind. We need to shut down our chattering mind because the chattering mind always occupies a large space. Silence in a regular interval can remove the clutters in our mind. Silence is a prayer and we can practice it ata particular time. Silence gives our mind more energy to think and remove the clutters. Silence conserves energy in our mind and it gives our mind more alertness.

Keep a smiling face. Smile is an ornament on our face. Smile is a great exercise for our facial muscles. It is a window to our communication. Start any conversation with a smile and see the impact. We forget our true self because of our ignorance. One smile can change a circumstance and bring favorable results to us. We stay connected to our true nature. So keep smiling all the time.

Get rid of the Clutter. Keep all your clutter at bay. Be it mental clutter or clutter at home. Clutters at home barricades our energy,so we need to clean the clutters on a regular basis to keep our energy level up at home. At the same time, our mental clutter needs to be cleaned everyday through forgiveness prayer. Initially, it seems to be an uphill task but regular practice can make it a habit and we can remove all the clutters from our life and make our life more vibrant and energetic.

Always practice the attitude of gratitude. In the morning we can practice Gratitude by maintaining a Gratitude Journal. You take a nice diary and start writing what you are grateful for,starting from the Universe to the people we come across in our life and their contribution in our life. Gratitude is the highest vibration in this universe and we need to practice it every day to rewire our mind. We can write "I am so happy and grateful to God for this amazing lovely wonderful awesome incredible successful life". In this way, we can write about the People, Material things, Essential things and many more that we are grateful for.

- ***Practice Giving and Receiving.*** We need to be a generous giver and an excellent receiver. If we are a generous giver then we can get more generosity from others. If we practice the art of giving then abundance would come to our life because whatever we give to the outside, it will come back to us in many folds and it is a Universal law.

- ***Maintain an abundance mentality.*** Everything is available in abundance in this Universe and the Universe is expanding. Abundance mentality can be developed. If we think that there is abundance in everything in our life and you have 100% faith in it then you can see that everything is available in this Universe in abundance. We need to drop the Scarcity mentality and develop an abundance mentality. It can be developed by using all the mind power tools, techniques and strategies.

- ***Pray for others.*** If we pray for others, our prayer can be listened. Whatever we send out,will come back to us. If you are generous and pray for others then the prayer will come back to you in many folds.
- ***Have unconditional love and acceptance for everyone, starting with self.*** Start self-love right now and it will reflect in the outer world. If you love yourself very much then you will receive the same love from others because it is the second powerful vibration in this Universe and whatever you send out will come back to you with many folds.
- ***Have faith in theUniversal power*** that it will always take care of you. Faith is very important in our life. If we have faith inthe Universal power then we can draw anything from it. There is a saying that Faith can move mountains. If we have doubts instead of faith then it will create a negative energy field outside us and we cannot accomplish our desired outcome.
- ***Undertake regular practice of meditation.*** Stay Connected to the Source. Regular connection with the source can give us power,we can stay connected

and draw resources from the source. Everything is there in the source. Only thing is to connect with it on a regular basis to draw the results.

- ***Practice Appreciation.*** Always appreciate people for their contribution to your life. Always appreciate their presence in your life. A small appreciation can change your relationship with others in a different way.

- ***Stay away from Negativity and Negative People.*** People who talk negative things can drain out your energy which can make you feel dull. You can feel your emotions when you are surrounded by negative people. At the same time, you can check your emotions when you are surrounded by positive people. You feel very good when you are surrounded by positive people and you urge to spend more time with them. You feel very uncomfortable when you are surrounded by negative people and you want to leave them as soon as possible.

- ***Do things that you love.*** Always give privilege to the work you love the most. Make a list of 20 things you love to do. Start doing all the listed work with full passion and see the results. If you are passionate about your work then work would no longer be work, you will just enjoy it.

- ***Regular exercise*** will keep your body fit. Yoga, Aerobics and dance can make your body vibrant. Walking 30 minutes for 5 days a week can keep many diseases at bay. Different breathing exercises can make our mind focused. In any adverse situation, only breathing exercise can help us to make our self stable. Through breathing exercise, we can slow down our mind to a great extent. If our mind is slow,calm and cool then our intellect awakes. Our body needs rest for at least 6-8 hours a day. Deprivation of sleep can have an adverse effect onour body and mind. Due to our sedentary lifestyle, we forget to take care of our body which is the most important asset in our life and we tend to abuse it. Every half an hour we need to move our body parts and we can do it easily at our workplace by stretching our body. Our body is the most precious thing in our life and it is like a motor car which needs proper maintenance at regular intervals. Intermittent fasting is the best way to detoxify our body. Our body consists of 70% water and to balance it we need regular consumption of water. Water and liquid consumption hydrate our body and flush out toxins from the body. Food habits have a great impact on our body. Raw fruits, vegetables and fiber diets are good for easy digestion. Our intestine is 6 meters long and it takes a long time to digest spicy and fried foods. Most of the sedentary lifestyle diseases are the result of mental stress and food. To maintain a healthy lifestyle, we need to maintain a routine in our life. Regular relaxation through meditation keeps our mind alert and focused which helps us to make the right decisions in our life.

- ***Our subconscious can't differentiate between the imagination and reality.*** So we need to act as if it is achieved. Start imagining the thing you need in life and visualize that it has been achieved. Enjoy the moment of achievement during visualization. Just visualize that it is happening right now in front of you. Our Subconscious mind can attract events, people and circumstances to make it a reality. The conscious mind needs to grab the opportunity as soon as it appears. Visualization is very effective in the morning after waking up and before retiring to the bed. In these times our mind is very slow and we enter into the Alpha state of consciousness which is the best time to connect to our subconscious mind. Active visualization with the feelings can instruct us to take inspired action to achieve the desired goals. Our subconscious mind brings people in our life that can help us achieve our goals. It pushes us to attend events where we can explore our way to achieve our goal.

Power Napis most useful when:

- You are tired at work or need to catch up on your sleep.
- You need to rest when driving long distances or traveling across time zones.
- Keeping yourself always charged and full of energy.

In these above conditions we need some energy-booster instantly. This power nap is a kind of relaxation for our mind. Only 20-30 minutes are good enough to rejuvenate ourselves. It can be done at your workplace as well. You only need some time with yourself. Sit quietly and take 10-20 deep breaths very slowly to calm down your mind. After 10 to 20 breaths just observe the breath for 5 minutes.Then come back to the body and give attention to all the body parts one by one from toes to head. Be aware of the surrounding. Slowly and gradually open your eyes. Just check how much energetic you will feel after this process.

CHAPTER 12

Corporate Hangover

Our mind is very much volatile in nature. It runs very fast. The speed of our mind is much more than that of light and sound. In our professional career we are always stuck and the amount of pressure managers take, they are rarely able to tolerate that pressure and hence, they carry it to their home. I called it the corporate hangover. This hangover cannot balance our both professional and personal life. We carry this corporate hangover all the time in our life. We are not accustomed to this pressure and our belief system always tells us that this is normal. In our corporate life, we always hear the term "Work Pressure" and we start believingafter listening to this term for several times. As we know that repetitive affirmations can directly go to our subconscious mind and start believing it as a reality. Human mind is designed in such a way that it absorbs things from the surroundings and coverts it as a strong belief. I used to do the same thing in my earlier days and suffered a lot. I could not understand it and carried it with me for a long time. It seemed that I was not prioritising my work and I suffered badly. Realization of our life and its purpose is very much needed to understand and make a plan for the future. We always search for our purpose butare lost somewhere and because of the pressure from the surrounding we do the job that we are not meant for. In this corporate world, we need to cool down our mind so that the intellect awakes and we take theright decision in any situation. We are the creator of our life and we make our destiny on our own. Our action will take us to our destination. Whatever you do, do it with 100%. We need to balance our life so that it would not affect our happiness. Being workaholic is a good thing because an idle mind is devil's workshop but at the same time, we need to balance our life. We don't understand our mind very well. We need to cut off from all of unimportant thingsat regular intervals. We can focus on a certain thing at a time and until and unless we finish it we should not move to the other work.Evidentally and scientifically, our mind works on one work at a time. We do multitasking every time and leave our work half done and jump to another work. This unfinished work cannot be done later because the momentum gets lost if we leave it in between. Our goal can be anything but we have to be consistent until we achieve it.Corporate commitment is very high and the work pressure is very high as well. We take everything on our head and we cannot control our mind because of the amount of work. In this pressure, we loose control and carry on with it for 24 hours which leads to stress and irritation. We need to calm down our mind and do our work as I mentioned that an agitated mind cannot open up our intellect and if our intellect is not awakened then we cannot make a right decision. Our mind controls everything and we need to program our mind in such a way that it is cool every time and in every situation. Self-talk is a very powerful tool to give command to our mind and align it. We need to understand that if mind conceives anything then it transforms into reality. Our childhood programming is responsible for our outcome because we shut the door when the opportunity comes and therefore, we get stuck. Our mind can receive any amount of information but what is dominant would work. So if our childhood programming is dominant then we can carry out our work that way. We are ears are fed with the statement that Job is very difficult;we need to work hard to get the salary etc.,these turn into powerful yet negative beliefs that start to dwell in our mind. Whenever we start a job we carry these beliefs with us and the jobs seem difficult and stressful. So, before giving any command to our mind, we need to think twice and analyze the old belief system.If anything toxic is there in our mind then we need to replace it with new affirmation. Self-affirmations are the most significant waysto rewire, restructure and recalibrate our mind. These affirmations can be in the present tense so that you can feel that it is happening right now. It can be for the workplace where you feel stressful and irritated. Initially, all the affirmations seem very unrealistic but we need to bypass our logical mind. Our logical mind always asks questions about anything and it gives a feeling that it is not realistic. There would be a contradiction inside the mind and we listen to our logical mind. We need to practice theseself-affirmations without any logic and if our logical mind comes in between,we need to continue with the affirmations so that after sometimes it accepts the command. It is a continuous process and we need to continue this process for a long time until and unless our mind accepts it.If we practice it ata regular interval then we can achieve it and can rewire our mind and belief system. Corporate hangover is very common nowadays because of our deadlines and commitments. Nowadays corporate are offering the work from home facility which is another reason for the hangover as there is a deficit of work-life balance.It creates issues inside our mind and acquires our personal space. Work-pressure in any organization is very high nowadays and people are unable to cope up with the pressure because of their lack of proper planning. Cross-functional activities sometimes create confusion and if people are not in sync with each other then the productivity would be decreased. Corporate productivity can be increased by relaxation techniques. Power Nap is the best relaxation techniques in the corporate. It gives instant energy to our mind and the productivity of our mind would increase significantly. If our mind is relaxed then our intellect awakes. We can focus our self in any work assigned to us. We can listen to a positive audio talk and practice positive affirmations. It will bring our mind back to the present moment. We are always thinking about the past and worried about the future and just forget the incredible present moment. We are not aware ofthe present moment. We need to enhance our awareness so that we can bring back our self in the present moment. The present moment is inevitable and we need to do our work with full awareness so that we can get the maximum results. Be aware of your surroundings and focus onyour work. Regular Relaxation and Meditation can bring back our life on the right track. We need to spend some time alone with the most beautiful person on this planet. We forget to care about our selfbecause of our over-commitment to others. Commitment to our body, mind and soul is the utmost priority and we cannot neglect it. If we give priority to our self then all the work will fall in place. We think that we need to change the outside but we forget the most important lessonin life that if we want to change the outside then we need to change ourselvesfrom the inside. Our outside is the exact mirror image of our inside, so we need to take care of our inside. If our inward journey is a roller-coaster ride then the outward journey is a roller-coaster ride as well. Modest lifestyle is the key to happiness. Desire is the seed of any creation but sometimes the desire takes away our happiness because we always strive for something which is only possible with consistent and persistent efforts. Our patience is very less,we accept failure as a permanent defeat and do not want to explore it further for any new possibilities. It is our mind which accepts or rejects the defeat. We need to equip our mind to accept the defeat as temporary and go forward to explore the new possibilities. Failure can teach us and give us the clue of possibilities. We need to explore opportunities in any adverse conditions. All the successful people do that and their mental state is unstoppable. All successful people accept their failure wisely and go ahead with the new zeal and dimension to defeat the failure. In my experience, if we train our mind with all the tools, techniques and strategies then we can accomplish outstanding results in our life. Our logical mind does not accept anything easily and puts a question mark in every situation. We need to nurture our Subconscious mind so that it can bring opportunities in front of us and helps us in achieving our goals. In our corporate life we need to set a desired goal and work on it. If we set a definite goal, we need to break it up into small goals and start working towards it. The first step towards our goal is vital. We need to take the first step after setting our goal and monitor our progress towards it. Our Personal and professional life has to be balanced and we cannot carry any work either way.

"A calm and modest life brings more happiness than the constant pursuit of success combined with constant restlessness."

- Albert Einstein

Major take away from this book:

- How to activate our inner self?
- Self-love and Self-care is explained.
- Importance of sound health.
- Human mind elaborated.
- Affirmations are the best tools to give command to our Subconscious mind.
- Anything is possible and everything is possible.
- Discovery of unstoppable mindset.
- Power of our Subconscious mind elaborated.
- Attitude of Gratitude and its power.
- Forgiveness prayer and its importance in our life.
- Self-introspection and to know yourself.
- Recalibration of our belief system.

- Our health is the most precious asset in our life.
- Relationship is the only key for happy and successful people.
- Relaxation and Meditation arethe food of our mind.
- Our true purpose of life.
- RespondVs React
- Listen to the inner voice.

For more information about our programs, kindly reach us@

mindcalinfo@gmail.com

info@mindcal.com

You can visit our website www.mindcal.com for details of our work.

Exercise

1) How do you connect to your Subconscious mind? Prepare a date-wise monthly chart for your activity on the Subconscious mind?

2) How many times you do Relaxation/Meditation in 24 hours? Monitor in a dairy and increase the duration of Meditation/ Relaxation slowly and gradually.

3) Check your purpose inlife! Make a list of 10 jobs you love to do. Search for your purpose in life.

____

____

____

____

4) Prepare a chart for your health. Monitor your exercise schedule, Meditation time and food intake on a weekly basis.

____

____

____

____

5) Do you practice Self-love or Self-care? How many times do you appreciate yourself with love in a day?

____

____

____

____

6) Prepare a Gratitude dairy for everything in life. Maintain it every day.

____

____

____

____

7) How many persons did you forgive today? Maintain a notebook and write down.

____

____

____

____

8) How many new relationships did you make today? Prepare a list of new relationships on a weekly basis.

____

____

____

____

9) How many times do you seek blessings from the Universe in a day? Monitor with awareness.

____

____

____

____

10) How many times you do affirmation on money energy in a day?

____

____

____

____

11) What are the 10 long term goals in your life?

____

____

____

____

12) What are the 10 goals in this financial year?

____

____

____

____

13) How many times do you need to connect to your vision board in a day? Prepare a chart and monitor every week.

____

____

____

____

14) How many mind tools are being explained in this book?

____

____

____

____

15) How many times do you take a Power Nap during the day? Please check the frequency and write down the timings in a chart.

____

____

____

____

16) Do yousometimes feel that you have a corporate hangover? Write down the steps to overcome the corporate hangover.

____

____

____

____

Made in the USA
Monee, IL
08 November 2026

67968597R00097